Time-Out in Child Behavior Management

About the Authors

Corey C. Lieneman, PhD, is a clinical child psychologist and assistant professor in the Department of Psychiatry at the University of Nebraska Medical Center. Her research and clinical interests lie in disruptive behavior disorders, autism spectrum disorder, and behavioral parent training for young children. She is level one trainer for Parent–Child Interaction Therapy (PCIT) International.

Cheryl B. McNeil, PhD, is a professor in the Department of Psychiatry at the University of Florida. She spent the previous 28 years of her career at West Virginia University. Dr. McNeil has coauthored many books, chapters, and over 150 research articles related to the importance of intervening early with young children displaying disruptive behaviors. Dr. McNeil is a global trainer for PCIT International and has disseminated PCIT to agencies and therapists in many states and countries, including Norway, New Zealand, Australia, Taiwan, Hong Kong, and South Korea.

Advances in Psychotherapy – Evidence-Based Practice

Series Editor
Danny Wedding, PhD, MPH, Professor Emeritus, University of Missouri–Saint Louis, MO

Associate Editors
Jonathan S. Comer, PhD, Professor of Psychology and Psychiatry, Director of Mental Health Interventions and Technology (MINT) Program, Center for Children and Families, Florida International University, Miami, FL
J. Kim Penberthy, PhD, ABPP, Professor of Psychiatry & Neurobehavioral Sciences, University of Virginia, Charlottesville, VA
Kenneth E. Freedland, PhD, Professor of Psychiatry and Psychology, Washington University School of Medicine, St. Louis, MO
Linda C. Sobell, PhD, ABPP, Professor, Center for Psychological Studies, Nova Southeastern University, Ft. Lauderdale, FL

The basic objective of this series is to provide therapists with practical, evidence-based treatment guidance for the most common disorders seen in clinical practice – and to do so in a reader-friendly manner. Each book in the series is both a compact "how-to" reference on a particular disorder for use by professional clinicians in their daily work and an ideal educational resource for students as well as for practice-oriented continuing education.

The most important feature of the books is that they are practical and easy to use: All are structured similarly and all provide a compact and easy-to-follow guide to all aspects that are relevant in real-life practice. Tables, boxed clinical "pearls," marginal notes, and summary boxes assist orientation, while checklists provide tools for use in daily practice.

Continuing Education Credits

Psychologists and other healthcare providers may earn five continuing education credits for reading the books in the *Advances in Psychotherapy* series and taking a multiple-choice exam. This continuing education program is a partnership of Hogrefe Publishing and the National Register of Health Service Psychologists. Details are available at https://www.hogrefe.com/us/cenatreg

The National Register of Health Service Psychologists is approved by the American Psychological Association to sponsor continuing education for psychologists. The National Register maintains responsibility for this program and its content.

Advances in Psychotherapy – Evidence-Based Practice, Volume 48

Time-Out in Child Behavior Management

Corey C. Lieneman
Department of Psychiatry, University of Nebraska Medical Center, Omaha, NE

Cheryl B. McNeil
Department of Psychiatry, University of Florida, Gainesville, FL

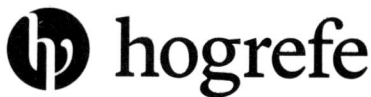

Library of Congress of Congress Cataloging in Publication information for the print version of this book is available via the Library of Congress Marc Database under the Library of Congress Control Number 2022950048

Library and Archives Canada Cataloguing in Publication
Title: Time-out in child behavior management / Corey C. Lieneman (Department of Psychiatry, University of Nebraska Medical Center, Omaha, NE), Cheryl B. McNeil (Department of Psychiatry, University of Florida, Gainesville, FL).
Names: Lieneman, Corey C., author. | McNeil, Cheryl Bodiford, author.
Series: Advances in psychotherapy--evidence-based practice ; v. 48.
Description: Series statement: Advances in psychotherapy--evidence-based practice ; volume 48 | Includes bibliographical references and index.
Identifiers: Canadiana (print) 20220475490 | Canadiana (ebook) 20220475601 | ISBN 9780889375093 (softcover) | ISBN 9781613345092 (EPUB) | ISBN 9781616765095 (PDF)
Subjects: LCSH: Timeout method. | LCSH: Discipline of children. | LCSH: Behavior modification.
Classification: LCC HQ770.4 .L54 2023 | DDC 649/.64—dc23

© 2023 by Hogrefe Publishing

www.hogrefe.com

The authors and publisher have made every effort to ensure that the information contained in this text is in accord with the current state of scientific knowledge, recommendations, and practice at the time of publication. In spite of this diligence, errors cannot be completely excluded. Also, due to changing regulations and continuing research, information may become outdated at any point. The authors and publisher disclaim any responsibility for any consequences which may follow from the use of information presented in this book.

Registered trademarks are not noted specifically as such in this publication. The use of descriptive names, registered names, and trademarks does not imply, even in the absence of a specific statement, that such names are exempt from the relevant protective laws and regulations and therefore free for general use.

The cover image is an agency photo depicting models. Use of the photo on this publication does not imply any connection between the content of this publication and any person depicted in the cover image. Cover image: © Antonio_Diaz – iStock.com

PUBLISHING OFFICES

USA:	Hogrefe Publishing Corporation, 44 Merrimac St., Suite 207, Newburyport, MA 01950 Phone 978 255 3700; E-mail customersupport@hogrefe.com
EUROPE:	Hogrefe Publishing GmbH, Merkelstr. 3, 37085 Göttingen, Germany Phone +49 551 99950 0, Fax +49 551 99950 111; E-mail publishing@hogrefe.com

SALES & DISTRIBUTION

USA:	Hogrefe Publishing, Customer Services Department, 30 Amberwood Parkway, Ashland, OH 44805 Phone 800 228 3749, Fax 419 281 6883; E-mail customersupport@hogrefe.com
UK:	Hogrefe Publishing, c/o Marston Book Services Ltd., 160 Eastern Ave., Milton Park, Abingdon, OX14 4SB Phone +44 1235 465577, Fax +44 1235 465556; E-mail direct.orders@marston.co.uk
EUROPE:	Hogrefe Publishing, Merkelstr. 3, 37085 Göttingen, Germany Phone +49 551 99950 0, Fax +49 551 99950 111; E-mail publishing@hogrefe.com

OTHER OFFICES

CANADA:	Hogrefe Publishing Corporation, 82 Laird Drive, East York, Ontario M4G 3V1
SWITZERLAND:	Hogrefe Publishing, Länggass-Strasse 76, 3012 Bern

No part of this book may be reproduced, stored in a retrieval system or transmitted, in any form or by any means, electronic, mechanical, photocopying, microfilming, recording or otherwise, without written permission from the publisher.

Printed and bound in the USA

ISBN 978-0-88937-509-3 (print) • ISBN 978-1-61676-509-5 (PDF) • ISBN 978-1-61334-509-2 (EPUB)
https://doi.org/10.1027/00509-000

Acknowledgments

I am incredibly grateful to my coauthor and the best mentor I have ever known, Dr. Cheryl McNeil, for her support and belief in me during the writing of this book and always. I am forever indebted to Cheryl for her expert training and professional guidance. Thank you to my husband, Casey, for his patience with this book project, as well as his unwavering encouragement as we navigated raising two young children during my graduate education. To my boys, Malachi and Benny, thank you for giving up your mom on Saturdays to make this book possible. Finally, I am thankful to my parents, Bill and Jody, for instilling in me the importance of hard work and education.

C.C.L.

Here is a loud shout out to all of the graduate and undergraduate students who have supported my work in the parent–child interaction therapy research lab over the years, as well as Dr. Sheila Eyberg who provided me with the gift of PCIT. I especially appreciate Erinn Victory who provided editorial comments on the first draft of this manuscript. I also want to thank my supportive husband, Dan, who held down the fort and provided moral support during the long absences needed for several book projects over the years. I also want to thank my sons, Danny and Will, who were willing to give up some "Mom time" so that I could pursue my academic dreams. Finally, hugs and thanks to my father, Otis, who encouraged me to excel in school and be the first in our family to attend college, as well as Jack and Debbie who have diligently helped our family through thick and thin.

C.B.M.

Preface

The concept of using time-out for child discipline has been a topic of attention for both researchers and the lay public for many decades. Sarah Vander Schaaff summarized the issues well in her 2019 *Washington Post* article about time-out researcher Dr. Arthur Staats entitled, "The Man Who Developed Timeouts for Kids Stands by His Now Hotly-Debated Idea" (Vander Schaaff, 2019). In the article, Vander Schaaf points out the controversies associated with this evidence-based approach for managing child disruptive behavior:

> Today, the merits of timeout are hotly debated. Some argue it is harmful, provoking feelings of isolation, abandonment and anxiety while doing little to teach self-regulation. Others maintain the discipline is effective and not only helps a child acquire self-control but also gives parents the opportunity to cool off and reduces yelling or physical abuse. Staats, now 95 and with two adult children, five grandchildren and two great-grandchildren, stands by his work from the early 1960s. 'TYM-OUT' proclaims his license plate. (Vander Schaaff, 2019)

Dr. Cheryl McNeil, one of the authors of this text, added to this *Washington Post* article by stating,

> When families and children are trained in the proper techniques for time-out – learning a system that involves creating a positive 'time-in' environment of parent–child interaction, explaining the rules of timeout in advance, using warning statements and consistent follow-through – children show great success… And it's a big flop if it's done without training and ineffectively. (Vander Schaaff, 2019)

In this book, we strive to flesh out the issues discussed in the *Washington Post* article, providing an overview of the research, as well as clinical details regarding time-out techniques. Our goal is to provide an even-handed description of the pros and the cons of time-out, with particular attention to empirical evidence and behavioral theory.

Contents

Acknowledgments v
Preface vi

1	**Description**	1
1.1	History of Time-Out	1
1.2	Defining Time-Out: Extinction or Punishment?	3
2	**Review of Time-Out Research**	6
2.1	Children With Attention-Deficit/Hyperactivity Disorder (ADHD)	8
2.2	Children With Autism Spectrum Disorder (ASD)	9
2.3	Children With Intellectual Disability/Cognitive Delay	10
2.4	Children With Internalizing Disorders	11
2.5	Child Trauma	11
2.6	Changing Caregiver Behavior	12
2.7	Child Compliance Training	13
2.8	Long-Term Outcomes of Child Behavior Management	14
2.9	Summary	14
3	**Using Time-Out: Developmental Age-Based Considerations**	15
3.1	Children Younger Than 24 Months	15
3.1.1	Managing Problem Behavior	15
3.1.2	Training Emotion Regulation and Self-Control	16
3.1.3	Compliance Training	17
3.2	Children Ages 2–10 Years	17
3.2.1	Cognitive Factors	18
3.2.2	Physical Factors	18
3.2.3	Social Factors	18
3.3	Children Ages 8–10 Years and Older	19
3.3.1	Managing Time-Out Refusal and Escape	20
3.3.2	Increasing Buy-In	20
3.3.3	Alternative Forms of Time-Out	22
4	**Diversity Issues**	25
4.1	Ethnic, Racial, and National Considerations	25
4.1.1	Minority Groups in the United States	26
4.1.2	International Views	27
4.1.3	Summary	28
4.2	Time-Out in Relation to Other Socioeconomic Factors	28
5	**Evidence-Based Programs Including Time-Out**	30
5.1	The Defiant Children Program	30
5.2	Family Interaction Training Program (FIT)	31
5.3	The Helping the Noncompliant Child Program	32

5.4	The Incredible Years Program	33
5.5	Parent–Child Interaction Therapy (PCIT)	34
5.6	The Kazdin Method (Formerly Parent Management Training)	34
5.7	Triple P – Positive Parenting Program	35
5.8	Summer Treatment Program	36
5.9	Parent Management Training – Oregon/ Generation PMT–O	37
5.10	Summary	37

6 Parameters of Time-Out ... 39

6.1	Verbalized Reason	40
6.2	Warning	40
6.3	Administration	41
6.4	Location/Type	42
6.4.1	Isolation Time-Outs	42
6.4.2	Exclusionary Time-Outs	42
6.4.3	Nonexclusionary Time-Outs	43
6.5	Duration	44
6.5.1	Brief Time-Outs	44
6.5.2	Longer Time-Outs	45
6.5.3	Contrast or Sequencing Effects	45
6.6	Schedule	46
6.7	Release From Time-Out	47
6.7.1	Time-Based Release	47
6.7.2	Behavior-Based Release	48
6.7.3	Time- and Behavior-Based Release	48
6.7.4	Comparing Release Contingencies	48
6.8	Escape	49
6.8.1	Escape *From* Time-Out	49
6.8.2	Escape *Through* Time-Out	50

7 Controversial Issues Related to Time-Out ... 52

7.1	Behavioral Parenting Approaches	52
7.2	Punishment	54
7.2.1	What Is Punishment?	55
7.2.2	Concerns With Punishment	55
7.3	Controversies Around Time-Out	59
7.3.1	Does Time-Out Cause Trauma and Physiological Harm?	60
7.3.2	Are There Other Negative Outcomes Associated With Time-Out?	61
7.3.3	Time-Out is Efficacious in Research, but Is It Effective in the "Real World"?	63
7.3.4	Does Time-Out Only Affect Immediate Behavior Problems?	64
7.3.5	Is Exclusively Positive Parenting Preferable to Time-Out?	65
7.3.6	Is Time-Out Widely Unacceptable?	67
7.4	Legal Issues	68
7.4.1	Modifications of Time-Out Procedures	68
7.4.2	Conclusion	69
7.5	Ethical Issues	69
7.6	Conclusion	70

8	**Parent–Child Interaction Therapy (PCIT) Time-Out as an Exemplar**	71
8.1	Introducing Time-Out	71
8.2	PDI Teach Session	72
8.2.1	Effective Commands	72
8.2.2	Effective Follow-Through	72
8.2.3	Return to Child-Directed Interaction	75
8.2.4	Planning for At-Home Practice	75
8.2.5	Planning for the First Discipline Coaching Session	76
8.3	First PDI Coaching Session	76
8.3.1	Preparing the Room	76
8.3.2	Preparing the Back-Up Space	77
8.3.3	Beginning the First Discipline Coaching Session	77
8.3.4	Teaching PDI to the Child	77
8.3.5	Coaching PDI	77
8.4	Gradual Roll-Out Approach	78
8.4.1	Time-Out for Other Behavior	79
8.5	Alternatives to Chairs, Back-Up Spaces, and Carrying Children	79
8.6	Conclusion	80
9	**Case Vignette**	81
9.1	Case Background	81
9.2	Treatment Plan and Goals	83
9.2.1	Treatment Session 1 (Relationship-Building Didactic & Coaching)	83
9.2.2	Treatment Session 2 (Relationship-Building Coaching & Differential Attention)	84
9.2.3	Treatment Session 3 (Relationship-Building Coaching & Discipline Didactic)	85
9.2.4	Treatment Session 4 (Compliance Training & Time-Out Coaching)	86
9.2.5	Treatment Session 5 (Compliance Training & Time-Out Coaching)	90
9.2.6	Treatment Session 6 (Compliance Coaching, House Rule, & Public Behavior Planning)	92
9.2.7	Treatment Session 7 (Follow-Up & Future Planning)	93
10	**Further Reading**	95
11	**References**	97
12	**Appendix: Tools and Resources**	110

Description

Time-out is short for time-out from positive reinforcement. In its most basic definition, time-out refers to "a period of time in a less reinforcing environment made contingent on a behavior" (Brantner & Doherty, 1983, p. 87). In other words, following a specific behavior, an individual is either moved to a less reinforcing environment or somehow limited in accessing reinforcement in the current environment. Time-out is typically used as a punishment procedure to discourage undesirable behavior. Although principles of time-out have been used in other arenas, for the purposes of this book we discuss time-out as it relates to child behavior management, predominantly in the United States.

Time-out is short for time-out from positive reinforcement

1.1 History of Time-Out

Some of the earliest discussions of time-out in the literature appear in studies of animal behavior from the 1950s (Ferster, 1958; Ferster & Skinner, 1957; Skinner, 1950). This research centered on training animals, such as pigeons and chimpanzees, to peck keys or press switches in order to access reinforcement in the form of food. When time-out from reinforcement was employed – animals no longer received food for responding (e.g., pressing keys or switches) – behavioral researchers discovered that rates of responding were impacted. This literature began to establish the study of time-out as a procedure in which animals' behavior mirrored behavior under conditions of other known forms of punishment. Most fundamentally, animals' responding for food decreased during periods of time-out. Relatedly, animals either responded more or less frequently before and after periods of time-out depending on how the experimenters arranged the contingencies (Ferster & Skinner, 1957).

Later, in the 1960s and 1970s, researchers began to generalize time-out procedures to applied settings. Children with disabilities demonstrating dangerous or destructive behavior were some of the first subjects to appear in the time-out literature. For example, Risley (1968) attempted to use time-out from social attention to decrease dangerous behavior (e.g., climbing bookshelves, hitting others) in a child diagnosed with autism. Similar time-out studies targeted self-injurious behavior, aggression, tantrums, elopement, and problems related to eating, sleeping, and toileting (Harris & Ersner-Hershfield, 1978). Subjects were often individuals with cognitive deficits, neurodevelopmental disabilities, or serious mental health diagnoses, especially those who were institutionalized. Time-out was employed as a less aversive alternative to

Time-out was first introduced to reduce dangerous or destructive behavior

popular methods of severe behavior management of the day, including corporal punishment, pharmacotherapy, and electric shock.

During this same period, time-out became broadly appealing as a practice for typically developing children. Behavioral learning theorists such as Gerald Patterson and Arthur Staats have been credited with introducing the concept of time-out as a component of childrearing (Patterson & White, 1969; Staats, 1971). However, the practice may have predated formal naming and study. Constance Hanf was another influential figure in the popularization of time-out as a parenting technique. Hanf developed a treatment program for improving parent–child interactions, which included time-out as a component of discipline (Hanf, 1969). Hanf's two-stage model went on to serve as a blueprint for many of the most evidence-based behavioral parent training programs in use today, including parent–child interaction therapy (PCIT; McNeil & Hembree-Kigin, 2010), Helping the Noncompliant Child (McMahon & Forehand, 2003), The Incredible Years (Webster-Stratton & Reid, 2017), Parent Management Training – Oregon (Dishion et al., 2016), and Triple P – Positive Parenting Program (Reitman & McMahon, 2013; Sanders, 1999). These programs, discussed further in Chapter 5, continue to support the effectiveness of time-out as a disciplinary strategy for children with disruptive behavior problems.

> **Psychologists Patterson and Staats introduced the concept of time-out in childrearing**

Along the same vein, various forms of time-out for child behavior management found their way into classroom settings in the 1970s. It was around this time that individual states began banning corporal punishment in schools (Forehand & McKinney, 1993). Student behavior such as tantrums, physical aggression, out-of-seat behavior, and general disruptiveness served as the first targets of classroom time-outs in the literature (Foxx & Shapiro, 1978; Porterfield et al., 1976). Researchers pioneered creative variants of time-out principles in public schools, daycare centers, camps, and special education settings for children aged 1–18 years.

> **Schools started implementing time-out in the 1970s**

Before the advent of time-out as a common disciplinary measure for children, other disciplinary methods like corporal punishment, defined as the intentional infliction of physical pain contingent upon target behavior, were more popular than they are today. Arthur Staats cited concerns with damaging the parent–child relationship through spanking as his motivation for creating time-out, a new technique he used with his own children in the 1960s (Vander Schaaff, 2019). In addition, the popularization of time-out was overlaid on historical changes in mainstream American parenting as outlined by Forehand and McKinney (1993): (1) Disciplinary standards became less strict and punishments less severe; (2) Parents shifted away from reliance on religious guidance and toward guidance from professionals (e.g., psychologists); (3) Focus on ethical and legal standards aimed at improving children's rights increased; and (4) Fathers became more involved in the social development of children.

> **Arthur Staats created time-out over concerns with spanking**

Changes in discipline practices have occurred worldwide as well. Corporal punishment of children is currently unlawful in more than 75 countries around the world, areas encompassing 77% of the world's child population (Global Initiative to End All Corporal Punishment of Children, 2020a). In contrast, corporal punishment by parents remains legal in the United States with at least 15 states still also allowing corporal punishment in public schools (Global

> **Corporal punishment is currently unlawful in 75 countries**

Initiative to End All Corporal Punishment of Children, 2020b). Still, the popularity and use of corporal punishment across demographics is declining. In one large longitudinal study, researchers found that American mothers across socioeconomic groups reported significant decreases in their use of spanking and significant increases in their use of time-out as disciplinary strategies from 1988 to 2011 (Ryan et al., 2016).

A key development during this time period was a policy statement from the American Academy of Pediatrics (AAP, 1998). Physical discipline has been associated with many negative outcomes such as poorer caregiver–child relationships, mental health problems, antisocial behavior, future abuse perpetration and victimization (Kazdin & Benjet, 2003). In turn, time-out has received strong empirical support (Kaminski et al., 2008). Based on this growing body of research, the AAP released their official position as discouraging corporal punishment and recommending nonphysical discipline, specifically naming time-out. More evidence behind the efficacy of time-out in comparison to other forms of discipline can be found in Chapter 2.

> **Physical discipline has many negative outcomes**
>
> **The AAP discourages corporal punishment**

From its origins in animal research 70 years ago, to its place as one of the most popular parenting strategies in use today, time-out has come a long way. As it originates from the field of behavior analysis, most time-out research and implementation has been conducted by behavior analysts or behavioral psychologists. As such, in the next section, we briefly define the behavioral underpinnings of time-out.

1.2   Defining Time-Out: Extinction or Punishment?

Researchers and behavioral learning theorists have disagreed as to whether time-out from positive reinforcement constitutes extinction, punishment, or both (Brantner & Doherty, 1983). Extinction, defined as the removal of a specific behavior's reinforcer, results in the decrease of a target behavior (Skinner, 1953). For instance, imagine a scenario in which a child's hitting behavior is maintained by escape. Each time a teacher assigns academic work, a student hits her and is sent to the principal's office, escaping the task. To implement extinction, the teacher would discontinue sending the child to the office (the reinforcer) immediately following the hitting behavior, insisting that the child complete the academic task. Hitting, in this scenario, should decrease because it is no longer being reinforced by escape.

> **Definition of extinction**

In addition to extinction, punishment is also a relevant concept. In behavioral terms, punishment is defined as a procedure in which some positive reinforcement is removed or an aversive stimulus is introduced following a target behavior; this procedure results in a reduction of a given behavior (Skinner, 1953). For example, caregivers may wish to reduce their children's hitting behavior toward siblings at home. A parent could remove access to a positive reinforcer (e.g., a favorite toy) or introduce an aversive stimulus (e.g., criticism) after the child hits to reduce the hitting behavior. The punishment procedure works because hitting is followed by the loss of reinforcement or exposure to an aversive stimulus. Given these definitions, the following arguments related to time-out can be posed.

> **Definition of punishment**

Time-out is an extinction procedure

Time-out is an extinction procedure. Let's say that a caregiver identifies the function of a child's screaming in the following scenario: A parent is busy working on the computer. Each time her child screams, the parent stops working, comes close to the child, and talks to them about the behavior. In this case, the screaming is reinforced or maintained by parental attention. After identifying this connection, the parent decides to extinguish the child's screaming by using time-out instead. With minimal attention from the mother, the child is sent to their room for 5 minutes each time they scream. If the screaming decreases because screaming is no longer being reinforced by parental attention, time-out can be considered an extinction procedure.

Time-out can be conceptualized as punishment

Applied or at least analyzed in a different way, time-out can be conceptualized as punishment. Using the same example, one could argue that the act of sending a child to their room is aversive. Similarly, being sent to one's room effectively removes the positive reinforcement of the original environment from the child. For example, in addition to social attention, the child may not be able to access food, television, or toys during the 5 minutes in their room alone. This removal of positive reinforcement is also considered punishment if it is followed by less screaming.

Time-out can both be punishment and extinction

Taken together, it might be argued that time-out can be both punishment and extinction, depending somewhat on circumstances. In our example, time-out functions as both. While it is possible to carry out a time-out procedure that can be considered purely punishment and not extinction or purely extinction and not punishment, the two are not *typically* mutually exclusive. Using the example of the child screaming to access parental attention, the mother may use time-out from her attention alone as a pure extinction procedure (and not punishment). In this scenario, she would continue to work on her computer, ignoring the screaming. The child would not be sent to their room, and therefore would not experience punishment through the imposition of a nonpreferred activity or removal of access to other privileges. This procedure is often referred to as planned ignoring or time-out from caregiver attention. Planned ignoring is effective at extinguishing problem behavior as long as the target behavior is not maintained by other factors. If, however, the child's screaming was simultaneously being reinforced by the mother's *and* sibling's attention, for example, then attempting to extinguish the behavior through a time-out from the mother's contingent attention alone would be less effective.

The same issues may apply to time-out procedures which employ only principles of punishment and not extinction. In our example, given the goal of decreasing screaming, the mother might carry the child to a time-out chair each time he screams. If the child gets up from the chair, she may scold him and carry him back to the chair repeatedly. In this case, the child is experiencing an aversive stimulus (e.g., criticism) and has been removed from other reinforcement (e.g., access to preferred activities, social attention from other family members). However, this time-out is not considered an extinction procedure because the stimulus reinforcing the screaming behavior, maternal attention, is not being removed.

Why does it matter if time-out works by punishment, extinction, or both? In short, understanding the behavioral underpinnings of time-out can help professionals and caregivers better harness the power of time-out under different circumstances. For instance, time-outs operating at least in part as punishment may be more effective in situations where the function of the behavior is unknown. Removing several sources of reinforcement (e.g., access to television and peer attention) by having a child leave the room, may decrease the problem behavior whether or not its function is related to TV or attention. This is particularly relevant when working with children for whom the reinforcing value of social attention may be decreased or unknown, for example children with autism spectrum disorder. In addition to social attention, sitting in a time-out chair for a few minutes effectively removes tangible reinforcement, increasing effectiveness of the procedure. On the contrary, when the function of problem behavior is known, time-outs operating purely through extinction may be less restrictive but still effective. For example, a child whose swearing is maintained by social attention alone can be allowed to remain in the original environment with access to other reinforcers as long as the swearing behavior itself is put on extinction (i.e., ignored) by surrounding peers and adults. The level of restriction used also has ethical implications, discussed further in Chapter 7.

Because components of extinction and punishment so often overlap, and both have utility in decreasing different cases of problem behavior, many time-out procedures employ both. Later in this book, we discuss specific parameters of time-out in general (Chapter 6), as well as unique formulations of time-out procedures within evidence-based treatment programs (Chapter 5 and Chapter 8). Time-out has been the topic of much research and debate over the past 70 years. Next, we provide a broad overview of the resulting literature.

2

Review of Time-Out Research

Time-out is recommended by the AAP as an effective disciplinary strategy

Time-out is considered a highly effective, evidence-based practice for child behavior management across the fields of child psychology and pediatrics. The American Academy of Pediatrics began recommending time-out as an effective disciplinary strategy in 1998 and continues to do so (AAP, 1998, 2018). The use of time-out for child behavior management has also been recognized by the American Psychological Association (APA; Novotney, 2012; Society of Clinical Child and Adolescent Psychology [SCCAP], 2017). These recommendations are built on scientific evidence. The time-out literature can be organized into two categories: (1) studies investigating the efficacy or effectiveness of time-out itself and (2) investigations of time-out as part of larger treatment packages. Although not an exhaustive review, this chapter describes much of the evidence around time-out in these two areas.

How has time-out been studied? The foundation of research investigating the efficacy and effectiveness of time-out as a tool for improving human behavior is made up of single-subject designs in applied behavioral research. In the 1960s, researchers found time-out to be useful in reducing a variety of child behavior problems (e.g., temper tantrums, thumb sucking, self-harm, undesirable mealtime behavior, disruptive classroom behavior, aggression, and even problematic consumption of alcohol; see Brantner & Doherty, 1983, for a review). More recently, researchers have continued to study the effects of time-out in both single-subject and group designs. The majority of the evidence clusters around the use of time-out to treat externalizing child behavior problems, most frequently aggression and noncompliance. Studies specifically investigating the effects of time-out often target populations of children at risk for or diagnosed with disruptive behavior disorders, conduct problems, attention-deficit/hyperactivity disorder (ADHD), and/or other disabilities.

Time-out has demonstrated effectiveness across settings

Regarding setting, time-out has demonstrated effectiveness in correctional programs, psychiatric treatment facilities, day-treatment programs, preschool and elementary school classrooms, summer camps, and the family home (Morawska & Sanders, 2011).

The field of BPT provides the most research evidence about time-out

The largest arena for studying time-out has been within behavioral parent training (BPT) research. Fittingly, the most effective, well-studied BPT programs all prescribe time-out. Of these, parent–child interaction therapy (PCIT; McNeil & Hembree-Kigin, 2010), Helping the Noncompliant Child (McMahon & Forehand, 2003), The Incredible Years (Webster-Stratton & Reid, 2017), Parent Management Training–Oregon (Dishion et al., 2016), and Triple P – Positive Parenting Program (Sanders, 1999) are some of the best supported. These treatments, and therefore time-out, are recognized as first-line treatments for disruptive behavior problems by a number of the most trusted

Treatments with time-out are first-line for disruptive behavior problems

leaders in mental health: the Substance Abuse and Mental Health Services Administration (SAMHSA, 2011), the American Psychological Association's Division 53: Society of Clinical Child and Adolescent Psychology (SCCAP, 2017), in the book *Evidence-Based Psychotherapies for Children and Adolescents* (considered to be the premier book on the topic; Kazdin, 2017), and in several large scale literature reviews of evidence-based psychosocial treatments for child and adolescent behavior problems (e.g., Kaminski & Claussen, 2017). The Centers for Disease Control and Prevention (CDC) also included time-out in their nationally disseminated program, *Essentials for Parenting Toddlers and Preschoolers* (CDC, 2019).

BPT programs use time-out in combination with other positive parenting strategies. Conceptually and empirically, time-out, without a contrast between conditions in and out of time-out, is less effective (e.g., Willoughby, 1970). Therefore, the treatment programs listed, and many others, incorporate components aimed at increasing positive caregiver–child interactions and desirable child behavior in addition to components aimed at decreasing undesirable child behavior, like time-out.

> Time-out is most effective when used in conjunction with high-quality time-in

In what ways do time-out and treatments that include it help children and families? Research supporting time-out has focused on several specific clinical topics. Most commonly, time-out independent of BPT has demonstrated effectiveness at reducing externalizing behavior problems (Kaminski et al., 2008). These problems can include physical aggression (e.g., hitting, biting, throwing objects), verbal aggression (e.g., yelling, name-calling), noncompliance (e.g., arguing, refusing to follow directions), and generally disruptive behavior (e.g., tantrums, interrupting). For example, Adams and Kelley (1992) found that time-out was effective at reducing sibling aggression. Donaldson and Vollmer (2011) demonstrated that time-out reduced screaming, persisting at a task when told to stop, and disrupting classroom activities in young children.

> Time-out reduces externalizing behavior problems

Similarly, BPT programs which include the use of time-out as a discipline strategy have also demonstrated effectiveness at reducing a variety of externalizing behavior problems, for instance, hyperactivity, aggression, and noncompliance (Comer et al., 2013; Eyberg et al., 2008). While BPT programs as a whole are important, time-out is a vital component. As an example, a study of the relative effectiveness of the two phases of PCIT (child-directed interaction and parent-directed interaction) demonstrated that the time-out component resulted in improvements in behavior problems from outside of normal limits to within normal limits (Eisenstadt et al., 1993). A meta-analysis of 77 parent training studies found that those treatments which included time-out were significantly more effective at reducing externalizing behavior problems than those programs that did not teach time-out (standardized mean difference effect sizes of 0.52 and 0.36, respectively; Kaminski et al., 2008).

> Parent training programs with time-out manage child behavior problems more effectively

If left untreated, children's externalizing behavior problems are likely to maintain or escalate over time (Broidy et al., 2003). For this reason, several treatment packages relying on time-out for discipline have been studied as prevention programs for future behavior problems. An adaptation of the Incredible Years program was found to be effective in preventing future conduct problems in Head Start students (Webster-Stratton, 2001). A Triple P prevention program administered through 12 television episodes, which advocated for the

> Treatment programs with time-out are more effective at preventing behavior problems

use of time-out, also demonstrated efficacy in preventing and decreasing child disruptive behavior (Sanders et al., 2000).

Time-out research is often conducted using disruptive behavior disorder samples. However, when opportunities for prevention are missed or are unsuccessful, children's behavior may later meet criteria for related disorders such as oppositional defiant disorder (ODD), conduct disorder, attention-deficit/hyperactivity disorder (ADHD), and/or another disruptive or antisocial disorder. Therefore, much of the time-out literature examines interventions for children within these populations. In children diagnosed with ODD, Nixon and colleagues (2003) showed clinically significant improvements in oppositional and conduct problems after treatment using time-out (i.e., both standard and abbreviated versions of PCIT). For children diagnosed with conduct disorder, McGuffin (1991) demonstrated the effectiveness of time-outs as brief as 5 minutes for decreasing aggression. As with externalizing behavior problems in general, if left untreated, children whose behavior meets criteria for a disruptive behavior disorder are more likely to maintain or develop greater psychopathology in the future (e.g., antisocial behavior, substance abuse, anxiety, depression; American Psychiatric Association [APA], 2013, Kaminski & Claussen, 2017). To mitigate these risks, time-out and interventions which employ it can be valuable tools for young children and their families with a variety of behavioral health diagnoses.

2.1 Children With Attention-Deficit/Hyperactivity Disorder (ADHD)

Research on time-out has also been conducted specifically in relation to children with ADHD. For example, Kapalka and Bryk (2007) showed that brief time-outs (i.e., 2–4 minutes) significantly decreased acting out behavior in boys diagnosed with ADHD. However, the majority of research on the use of time-out with ADHD child samples can be found within larger treatment programs that employ time-out. Authorities such as the CDC and the American Academy of Pediatrics (AAP) specifically recommend BPT (which often incorporates time-out) as a first line treatment for children with ADHD (CDC, 2022; Wolraich et al., 2019). In fact, the AAP recommends BPT even for children younger than age 5 who demonstrate symptoms of ADHD but are too young to be diagnosed (Wolraich et al., 2019). These recommendations draw on studies such as the Multimodal Treatment of ADHD study, a large, randomized clinical trial, which provided evidence that a combination of intensive behavioral intervention and medication or medication alone produced the best outcomes for children with ADHD. In some outcome measures (e.g., aggressive behavior, oppositional behavior, parent–child interactions), the combination of behavioral treatment and medication was superior to medication alone (The MTA Cooperative Group, 1999).

Relatedly, the Children's Summer Treatment Program (described further in Chapter 5) is an evidence-based program for children with ADHD which incorporates time-out. Both STP and its time-out procedure in particular have been shown to be effective in improving child conduct problems, interrupting, compliance, negative verbalizations, and school seatwork completion in children diagnosed with ADHD and disruptive behavior problems (Chronis et al., 2004; Fabiano et al., 2004).

2.2 Children With Autism Spectrum Disorder (ASD)

Externalizing behavior problems are also prevalent in populations of children diagnosed with other psychological disorders. As many as 53% of children with autism spectrum disorder (ASD), for example, demonstrate aggressive and/or disruptive behavior problems (Mazurek et al., 2013). In ASD, behavior problems often stem from communication deficits, difficulties adapting to change, and general emotion regulation challenges. In the past, researchers and treatment developers discouraged the use of time-out for individuals with ASD. Because social attention is less reinforcing for individuals with ASD, the idea of removing it as a consequence through time-out was thought to be ineffective. Many treatment models and their large-scale research have excluded children with autism based on this premise.

Empirical evidence on the topic is mixed. Raising further concerns for the use of time-out with individuals with ASD, Solnick and colleagues (1977) actually found time-out to be a *reinforcer* for one autistic child's tantrums because the time-out gave her the chance to engage in self-stimulatory behavior. To ameliorate this problem, other researchers found a *movement suppression time-out* in which children were physically prevented from engaging in automatically reinforcing body movements, to be effective (Rolider & Van Houten, 1985). In recent years, research has shown that traditional time-out procedures and treatment packages that include it *are* effective at reducing undesirable behavior for children with milder presentations of ASD (e.g., level 1 and level 2 for social communication; Lieneman et al., 2019; McNeil et al., 2018).

Two factors are likely to contribute to time-out effectiveness in children with ASD. First, as with all children, the environment from which the child is removed during time-out must be reinforcing. This means maximizing desirable and minimizing undesirable stimuli. For this reason, BPT programs focus on increasing the reinforcement value of caregiver attention. Tailored to children with ASD, techniques may include engaging with children in selected restricted and repetitive behavior. For these children, ensuring that social attention is reinforcing not only helps the parent–child relationship but increases the effectiveness of time-out. Likewise, the environment outside of time-out should match the child's stimulation needs. For instance, if a child with ASD is overstimulated by the noise, chaos, and social demands of a school cafeteria, time-out could be experienced as a pleasant escape. Time-out would not be likely to reduce problem behavior in this scenario. In fact, removal of children to a calmer, less demanding environment (e.g., principal's office) following problem behavior often makes the problem behavior worse over time. As such, settings in which a child with ASD is initially comfortable are better suited for time-out implementation.

Second, time-out for children with ASD is more likely to be effective when it limits access to social and nonsocial reinforcement. Lack of access to preferred tangibles (e.g., iPad), edibles (e.g., snacks), preferred sensory stimulation (e.g., music), and activities (e.g., running) during time-out may serve to discourage future problem behavior whether or not the removal of social attention has any impact. (See the discussion of extinction vs. punishment in Chapter 1). Therefore, forms of time-out that only employ differential attention for undesirable behavior alone may be less effective than a broader removal of access to other reinforcers in the environment, especially for children with ASD.

> **Time-outs that limit social AND nonsocial reinforcement may be more effective for children with ASD**

2.3 Children With Intellectual Disability/ Cognitive Delay

As discussed in Chapter 1, at its inception, time-out research predominantly used children with pervasive developmental disorders or what we would call intellectual disability today. Therefore, much of the scientific literature relates to the use of time-out for effective behavior management in these populations (Brantner & Doherty, 1983). More recently, some concerns have been raised about the use of time-out with individuals displaying lower functioning who may not understand simple instructions. Although time-out can be effective for these individuals, many caregivers and therapists are understandably uncomfortable with delivering a consequence to a child who does not fully understand the contingencies beforehand. For this reason, adaptations to time-out may be helpful. For example, therapists and caregivers may wish to incorporate a time-out readiness phase (i.e., compliance training with physical prompting as the consequence for noncompliance) before beginning to use time-out with children who have difficulty understanding more than a few simple instructions (McNeil et al., 2018).

> **Adaptations of time-out may be helpful for these children**

To ensure that children understand expectations before introducing any consequences, such as time-out for noncompliance, the following strategies may be helpful:

> **Strategies to ensure child comprehension of time-out**

1) Use simple language (e.g., "[child's name] close door.").
2) Model how to follow the instruction.
3) Role play what will happen following compliance (e.g., praise) and noncompliance (e.g., time-out procedure). Consider using a doll, stuffed animal, or another family member to act as the child.
4) Following instruction, use hand-over-hand guidance to help the child complete the task, followed by specific praise for compliance. Hand-over-hand guidance involves the adult placing their hands over the child's and guiding the child's hand through the activity as it is being taught.
5) Incorporate visual supports to introduce the steps involved with following instructions and steps to time-out (the *PCIT Time-Out Flip Book* is a great resource; Masse & Girard, n.d.)
6) Read social stories with the child. These are simple picture books detailing the steps to social routines (e.g., following instructions, time-out).
7) Give specific praise for following instructions throughout the day. This can help children start to recognize the steps to compliance in a positive

way. For a more structured approach, the tell, show, try again, guide sequence (Girard et al., 2018) is a particularly useful time-out alternative for very young children (under 2 years) and those with autism and lower receptive language abilities.

2.4   Children With Internalizing Disorders

While most research involving time-out includes children diagnosed with disabilities and disruptive behavior disorders, children with internalizing diagnoses such as anxiety and mood disorders can also benefit. Although these children experience many symptoms privately (e.g., low mood, negative cognitions, worry), anxious and depressed children are more likely than anxious and depressed adults to demonstrate irritability. Highly irritable or anxious children may display emotional outbursts and engage in avoidance, which can contribute to problems with compliance and disruptive behavior. For example, children with generalized, social, or separation anxiety often refuse to attend school or interact socially with peers. Similarly, children diagnosed with depression or other mood disorders may have low motivation to engage in tasks of daily living.

Children with internalizing disorders benefit from time-out

Time-out and treatments incorporating time-out have been employed to increase compliance and decrease problem behavior in children with anxiety and mood disorders (Puliafico et al., 2012). Larger treatment packages promoting positive caregiver–child interactions, emotion regulation, and coping skill development in addition to time-out, have demonstrated decreases in depression (Lenze et al., 2011) and anxiety (Chronis-Tuscano et al., 2015; Pincus et al., 2008). It is important to note that children are not directly put into time-out for exhibiting anxious or depressive behavior. On the contrary, caregivers in these programs learn to differentiate anxious and depressive behavior from purely defiant behavior, and time-out can be employed with the latter.

Treatment incorporating time-out has demonstrated decreases in child depression and anxiety

While most evidence supports the use of time-out for children with depression and anxiety, one study seemed to contradict these findings. In a cross-sectional survey of parenting practices, data suggested that frequency of time-out usage was positively associated with mother-reported but not self-reported child anxiety symptoms (Gershoff et al., 2010). This finding highlights the importance of avoiding overuse of time-out (see Chapter 6) and administering time-out in a context of other positive parenting strategies (see Chapter 5).

Importance of avoiding overuse of time-out

2.5   Child Trauma

The use of time-out in relation to concerns for child trauma has been hotly debated by clinicians and researchers alike. Currently, there are no data to suggest that time-out can traumatize or re-traumatize children. In fact, the Kauffman Best Practices Project to Help Children Heal From Child Abuse

There is no data that suggest that time-out traumatizes children

(2004) recommended three evidence-based treatments for children who had experienced abuse and neglect: trauma-focused cognitive behavioral therapy (TF-CBT; Cohen et al., 2010); Alternatives for families: A cognitive behavioral therapy (AF-CBT; Kolko et al., 2018); and parent–child interaction therapy (PCIT; Eyberg & Funderburk, 2011). In all three programs, among other components (e.g., developing a trauma narrative, psychoeducation about trauma, relationship building), a portion of therapy is devoted to caregiver training in child behavior management skills, and time-out can explicitly be taught.

> **Treatment with time-out reduces externalizing behaviors in children with trauma**

In comparison to TF-CBT and AF-CBT, PCIT devotes a much larger proportion of treatment to child behavior management and time-out. PCIT has demonstrated improvements in child externalizing behavior and caregiver–child relationships for families with histories of abuse and neglect (Batzer et al., 2018). Only one PCIT study has investigated treatment effects in direct relation to existing trauma symptoms. Pearl and colleagues (2012) used PCIT to treat children with various trauma histories (e.g., physical abuse, neglect, medical treatments, exposure to disasters, witnessing death). Results showed significant decreases across trauma symptoms, including posttraumatic related arousal, anxiety, intrusion, and dissociation, following intervention. Similarly, Akin and colleagues (2019) studied outcomes for foster children with histories of abuse and neglect following participation in Parent Management Training – Oregon (which uses time-out) with the addition of trauma-related content. Results revealed significant decreases in child socio-emotional problems (e.g., internalizing, mood, and thinking problems and self-harm) that may be associated with trauma.

> **Treatment with time-out may reduce trauma symptoms**

With the exception of BPT models, little research has examined the impact of time-out on trauma symptoms, and *no research* has found that time-out causes or exacerbates trauma symptoms. In the next section, we describe the evidence supporting time-out as a preventative measure against future trauma.

2.6 Changing Caregiver Behavior

> **Time-out improves caregiver behavior**

In addition to treatment of child behavior problems, time-out is also effective at improving caregiver behavior. Arguably one of the most important evidence-based uses of time-out is in the prevention of child abuse. In groundbreaking research, Chaffin and colleagues (2004; 2011) showed that PCIT effectively reduced recidivism rates for parents with histories of perpetrating child abuse in comparison to a standard community-based program. The authors posited that caregiver–child dyads are most vulnerable to instances of child abuse when engaged in a coercive cycle (Chaffin et al., 2004). The coercive family process, as conceptualized by Patterson (1979), is a negative caregiver–child interaction cycle in which both parties learn to escalate their own behavior in response to the other, creating a habitual power struggle. The coercive family cycle often develops around caregiver demands and attempts at discipline. Therefore, evidence of reduction in child abuse recidivism rates may be attributed in large part to the structure and consistency of the time-out procedure.

> **The coercive family process/cycle involves a habitual power struggle**

Caregivers trained in a structured time-out procedure are better able to respond calmly and consistently during interactions that may have historically become aggressive. In fact, PCIT, specifically the discipline phase of PCIT which includes time-out, has been associated with significant improvements in emotion regulation for caregivers and children, above and beyond improvements demonstrated during the relationship-building phase of treatment alone (Lieneman et al., 2020).

Caregivers learn to respond calmly and consistently

Parenting stress is another important factor to consider when targeting child abuse potential. Because higher levels of parenting stress are linked with higher potential for child abuse (Abidin, 1995), and BPT programs using time-out have demonstrated effectiveness in reducing parenting stress (Lieneman et al., 2020; Whitacre et al., 2020), stress reduction may be another mechanism for decreasing the likelihood of future perpetration.

Treatments with time-out demonstrate improvements in emotion regulation and parenting stress

2.7 Child Compliance Training

Throughout our discussion of time-out effectiveness, child compliance is a common thread. Noncompliance is considered a disruptive behavior for which time-out is a highly effective treatment (Eyberg et al., 2008; Kaminski et al., 2008). Though not limited to compliance training, time-out's effectiveness in every one of the previously described domains can be attributed at least in part to improved child compliance. In the treatment of disruptive behavior disorders, caregivers can use time-out to motivate completion of tasks without argument, an especially important treatment goal for children with oppositional defiant disorder (ODD) and conduct disorder. Alternatively, time-out can be used to motivate compliance with instructions to engage in positive behavior (e.g., walking quietly) which is incompatible with disruptive behavior (e.g., stomping).

Time-out is a highly effective treatment for noncompliance

Beyond disruptive behavior problems, child compliance is foundational in improving behavior for children with ADHD, anxiety, and mood disorders. Many evidence-based interventions for these disorders (e.g., exposure and response prevention, medication management) are only effective if children cooperate with treatment. This may mean motivating task completion for children with ADHD, exposure for children with anxiety, behavioral activation for children with depression, and medication adherence for all three. Of course, these tasks should rely heavily on positive reinforcement strategies. However, if basic child compliance and instructional control are established, treatment outcomes are more likely to be positive.

Compliance is foundational in improving child behavior

As such, time-out and its role in compliance training can be seen as a gateway intervention to a host of positive outcomes. Compliance can positively impact daily functioning (e.g., hygiene, school attendance), complementary services (e.g., speech therapy, occupational therapy), and social engagement (e.g., sports teams, positive caregiver-child relationships). This is not to say that time-out is necessary or sufficient in motivating child compliance. However, because time-out is an evidence-based strategy for improving compliance, and child compliance is such an integral part of healthy development, the connection among time-out and a broad range of positive child outcomes is relevant.

2.8 Long-Term Outcomes of Child Behavior Management

Time-out has lasting effects at follow-up

While the evidence of short-term effectiveness in child behavior management is clear, what does the literature say about long-term outcomes? Studies of time-out have demonstrated lasting effects at follow-up. For instance, Lavigueur and colleagues (1973) showed lasting effects of time-out at a 2-year follow-up assessment. Time-out was more effective than differential attention alone at decreasing disruptive behavior, effects which even generalized to a sibling.

More research has reported sustained improvements in child behavior following participation in BPT programs involving time-out. For example, Baum and Forehand (1981) found that child externalizing behavior improvements had maintained at 1–4.5 years posttreatment. Similarly, Hood and Eyberg (2003) showed that reductions in child disruptive behavior problems had maintained or even continued to decrease over the 3–6 years following initial improvements with PCIT. Further, in a 14-year follow-up of their BPT program which incorporated time-out, Long and colleagues (1994) found no differences at follow-up between young adults who had been referred as young children for behavior problems and a matched sample of nonclinical controls.

No evidence of long-term negative impacts of time-out

Finally, we found no evidence of long-term negative impacts of time-out or BPT packages that use a time-out procedure. To investigate whether or not time-out as an individual technique had negative long-term impacts, Knight and colleagues (2020) analyzed data from the Early Head Start Research and Evaluation study, which followed children from ages 0–3 years through the fifth grade. This study compared families who did and did not report using time-out of their own accord; time-out was not associated with any formal intervention efforts. No significant between-groups differences were found on the variety of outcomes measured including child internalizing (e.g., anxiety, depression), externalizing (e.g., aggression, rule-breaking), and caregiver–child relations (e.g., positivity toward parents). Separate analyses revealed greater externalizing problems for children whose caregivers had used physical discipline measures (Knight et al., 2020). Taken together, these studies demonstrate that there is no evidence of long-term detrimental effects associated with the use of time-out; however, time-out alone is not a guaranteed fix for all child behavior management problems.

2.9 Summary

Time-out is an evidence-based strategy for child behavior management. Much of its empirical support comes from the BPT literature. Time-out is an effective treatment for child externalizing behavior (e.g., aggression, disruptive behavior, noncompliance). Research also supports the use of time-out for a variety of other presenting concerns and populations. There is no available evidence of long-term negative outcomes related to time-out.

3

Using Time-Out: Developmental Age-Based Considerations

In this chapter, we discuss important considerations to determine whether standard or modified time-out procedures are appropriate based on the child's developmental age. Throughout this chapter, unless otherwise noted, we refer to child age based on what would be expected for a typically developing child. Most evidence-based parenting interventions recommend time-out as appropriate for children beginning around 2 years of age with use up through about 7–10 years of age (HNC, McMahon & Forehand, 2003; PCIT, Eyberg & Funderburk, 2011; Triple P, Sanders et al., 2003). We address considerations surrounding the use of time-out with children younger than this standard age range (i.e., infants and toddlers), children within the typical 2–7- to 10-year-old range, and children older than this age range. Specific modifications and alternatives to time-out are also described.

Time-out is often recommended for children ages 2–10 years

3.1 Children Younger Than 24 Months

Simply put, time-out is not typically recommended for children with abilities below those of a typically developing 2-year-old because other milder strategies are usually sufficient. However, there are special cases where forms of time-out have demonstrated effectiveness with children as young as 4 months of age (feeding disorders, Larson et al., 1987; dangerous behavior, Mathews et al., 1987). Still, for most younger children, the goals of time-out – managing problem behavior, teaching emotion regulation and self-control, and training compliance – can be accomplished through other approaches. We review developmental considerations related to these goals and offer suggestions about how to accomplish them without time-out.

Milder discipline strategies are usually sufficient for young children

3.1.1 Managing Problem Behavior

First, because infants and toddlers are small and have limited physical and cognitive abilities, environmental interventions are sufficient for managing and even preventing problem behavior in most situations. This may mean moving the child, or objects in relation to the child, to facilitate the desired behavior. For instance, a child may be picked up and placed in a crib when it is time to sleep or in a highchair when it is time to eat. Infants and toddlers can be carried easily from one location to the next. They can be physically removed

Environmental interventions are usually sufficient

from negative interactions with others or dangerous environments. Similarly, objects in the environment can be moved to places where infants and toddlers cannot access them, either because they cannot get at them physically or do not understand how to gain access. For example, caregivers can keep food on a high shelf to prevent children from eating unhealthy snacks, lock outside doors to keep children from leaving the home unattended, or turn off toys and electronics to discontinue their use.

3.1.2 Training Emotion Regulation and Self-Control

Common causes of infant and toddler disruptive behavior

Second, the goals and strategies involved with training emotion regulation and self-control are different for children younger than 2 years than for older children. Disruptive behavior in infants and toddlers often stems from immaturity in communication skills, cognitive abilities, learning histories, and independent emotion regulation capacities (Cole et al., 2004; Diamond, 2002). This makes time-out unnecessary in many circumstances for very young children.

Consider the following scenario. A parent and child wait in the checkout line at a grocery store. The child grabs a candy bar from the shelf and attempts to put it in his mouth. The parent says, "no," and puts the candy bar back on the shelf. In response, the child screams, cries, and tries to retrieve the candy bar. This scenario can be interpreted and managed very differently depending on the age of the child involved. If the child is 12 months old, he may not understand why he cannot have the candy bar and feel so upset by this turn of events that he breaks down crying. Without more sophisticated abilities to discuss the situation with his caregiver, the coping skills to manage his emotions independently, or the learning history and cognitive abilities to understand why this behavior is not allowed in this circumstance, the child's tantrum could be considered a reasonable response to a frustrating event. In this case, time-out might be inappropriate.

On the other hand, imagine if this child is a typically developing 7-year-old. He likely has the language abilities to communicate his concerns with his caregiver and the cognitive abilities and learning history to understand why he is not allowed to take and eat the candy bar. Further, he is more likely to have developed alternative emotion regulation strategies like distracting himself instead of throwing a tantrum. Even if the child is disappointed by the denial of access to the candy bar, he may cry but would be less likely to scream or defy the caregiver by trying to retrieve the candy.

If, however, the 7-year-old engages in a defiant tantrum, despite having adequate cognitive and communication abilities, this behavior may be better understood through a pattern of negative caregiver–child interactions. Other factors such as negative attention-seeking, a history of defiance and noncompliance, and perhaps engagement in the coercive process are more likely to explain this behavior. For more information about the coercive family process (Patterson, 1979), see Chapter 2. Similarly, older children exhibiting these negative behaviors often experience related deficits in emotion regulation (Gilliom et al., 2002). Appropriately, preschoolers and elementary aged children have demonstrated improved development of emotion regulation and self-control following limit setting with time-out (Lieneman et al., 2020).

Conversely, infants and toddlers are less likely than older children to have learned behavior problems that involve manipulative or coercive interactions reinforced through dysfunctional caregiver-child interactions. Their limited emotion regulation abilities are normative, as independent emotion regulation skills develop with age (Cole et al., 2004). Therefore, emotion regulation goals for infants and toddlers revolve around coregulation with a caregiver rather than developing more independent skills. As such, time-out is less appropriate for infants and toddlers who more often require the physical and emotional support of a caregiver to regulate. This may occur through using a soothing tone of voice, holding the child, offering a comforting touch, redirecting the child with other activities, or moving the child to another environment (Girard et al., 2018).

Infants and toddlers require more physical and emotional support

3.1.3 Compliance Training

Third, compliance training for infants and toddlers can be highly effective without the use of time-out. As their receptive language, cognitive, and motor abilities develop, caregivers can work with infants and toddlers to shape their abilities to follow simple instructions. By the same token, lack of follow-through with simple instructions by children in this age range should be interpreted with caution. Noncompliance may be attributed to lack of understanding, limited focus, or underdeveloped motor skills. As such, punitive consequences like time-out for noncompliance are often inappropriate and ineffective for infants and toddlers.

Caregivers can shape children's abilities to follow instructions

In younger children, lack of understanding and focus may contribute to noncompliance

Again, because of less sophisticated cognitive abilities and greater reliance on caregivers, infants and toddlers can be more easily motivated to comply without the use of negative consequences. Developmentally appropriate caregiver instructions are already quick and relatively simple (e.g., point to your nose) as compared with those appropriate for older children (e.g., clean your room). Positive reinforcement alone may be sufficient motivation, for example, enthusiastic clapping from the caregiver. If, however, the infant is distracted or does not understand the instruction, caregiver modeling and guided compliance are effective strategies. A sequence for compliance training with infants and toddlers without the use of time-out is outlined in the parent–child interaction therapy (PCIT) – toddlers model (Girard et al., 2018).

Positive reinforcement may be sufficient motivation for young children

3.2 Children Ages 2–10 Years

While there are exceptions, the majority of empirical evidence and theoretical support for the use of time-out for behavior management implicates children in the early preschool through late elementary school age range (i.e., 2–10 years). A variety of cognitive, physical, and sociocultural factors impacting children in this age range contribute to time-out effectiveness.

Usually time-out is recommended for children ages 2–10 years

3.2.1 Cognitive Factors

Understanding the basics of cause and effect develops at around 24 months

Receptive communication skills should be established before using time-out

Starting at the developmental age equivalent of about 24 months, most children are able to understand verbal instructions and the basics of cause and effect related to these instructions. Once toddlers can understand these basics of receptive communication, they are ready to learn through positive reinforcement for following instructions and removal of positive reinforcement (e.g., time-out) for noncompliance. Throughout the preschool, early-, and middle-childhood years, caregivers may continue to use time-out effectively to promote desirable behavior.

3.2.2 Physical Factors

Physically removing a child from a reinforcing environment is useful for smaller children

There are several reasons time-out can be such an effective method of discipline for this age range (i.e., ages 2–10) as compared with older children. First, and most simply, younger children are easier to carry and move. If removing the child from a reinforcing environment is a key component of time-out, then the ability to physically move a noncompliant child is a major advantage. Older and larger children require more physical strength and sometimes more careful planning by caregivers when attempting to execute time-out. Not only are younger children lighter, making them easier to lift, but their physical abilities are less developed. They cannot kick as hard, run away as quickly, or cling to things such as door frames as tightly to prevent themselves from going to time-out.

3.2.3 Social Factors

Caregivers are the source of a great deal of young children's reinforcement

Caregivers can motivate desirable behavior through reinforcement

Caregivers of children ages 10 and younger serve as powerful social and emotional influencers in their children's lives. During the preschool and elementary school years, caregivers are the source of a great deal of children's reinforcement. Caregivers provide physical affection, food, toys and other preferred tangibles, financial support, social interaction and attention, and access to and involvement in preferred activities. In turn, caregivers of young children are the keepers of access to reinforcement in most contexts. Therefore, caregivers can strategically deliver and withhold reinforcement to motivate desirable behavior from their children. Additionally, the caregiver–child bond is typically the most significant relationship in young children's lives. Peers and romantic partners do not yet wield as much social influence as they do in adolescence. Finally, the majority of young children's time is spent in proximity to their caregivers, either at home, school, or childcare centers. This provides ample opportunities for caregivers to enact effective behavior management strategies.

Self-control and emotion regulation skills are enhanced through time-out

Equally important is a caregiver's responsibility to help children develop socially and emotionally in the context of a supportive relationship. When used within a caregiver–child relationship built on consistent positive interactions, time-out helps children learn vital skills in emotion regulation and self-control (Kapalka & Bryk, 2007; Lieneman et al., 2020). Using time-out, caregivers can motivate their children to behave in ways conducive to healthy development. Skills like impulse control, compliance with directives from authority figures, and emotion regulation can be cultivated using time-out. Stronger skills in these areas are associated with greater success academically and in relationships (Trentacosta & Shaw, 2009), as well as with fewer problems related to criminal activity, mental and physical health problems, and substance abuse (APA, 2013; Trentacosta & Shaw, 2009).

3.3 Children Ages 8–10 Years and Older

Most evidence-based behavioral parent training programs recommend the use of traditional, location-based time-out (e.g., chair time-out) for children no older than about 7–10 years of age (HNC, McMahon & Forehand, 2003; PCIT, Eyberg & Funderburk, 2011; Triple P, Sanders et al., 2003). Next, we discuss important factors to consider when determining whether a child has matured beyond the appropriate developmental level for effective use of a standard therapeutic time-out (as described in Chapter 8). We also introduce several methods for tailoring or adapting time-out to fit the needs of older children. Finally, effective alternatives to time-out that can be used as children transition out of the appropriate age range for time-out are illustrated.

Traditional, location-based time-outs (e.g., chair time-outs) work well for children younger than 8–10 for a variety of reasons. Vice versa, managing problem behavior in older children presents some unique challenges.

First, negative patterns of behavior are typically more established in older children and their families. Older children are more likely to have developed sophisticated strategies for opposing and escaping caregivers' directives. While a 3-year-old may cry or throw herself on the floor to avoid getting into the car to go to school, a 10-year-old might falsely describe feeling sick to avoid going to school. It is easy to see why a time-out could be a simpler, more clear-cut strategy for parents to employ with the younger child in this scenario. Similarly, older children have likely had more experience with being reinforced through escaping caregiver demands or countercontrol (Skinner, 1953) over the years. In turn, caregivers and older children have had more opportunities to become entrenched in the coercive process (Patterson, 1979).

Older children may develop sophisticated strategies for escape and noncompliance

Histories of escape and countercontrol contribute to the coercive process

Second, as children get bigger, stronger, and more mature, their strategies for escaping traditional time-out typically become more difficult to manage. When a child is 10 years old and unwilling to go to time-out, he is usually better equipped to escape it by running away, becoming aggressive, or engaging in more sophisticated verbal arguments than when he was 2 years old. Similarly, a 10-year-old child can less easily be made to stay in a time-out chair or be moved to a back-up space by a caregiver. Size and mobility should be considered when working with families whose children are too large to carry or whose caregivers have limited physical abilities. Especially with families of older children, health and safety risks should be carefully discussed (Forcino et al., 2019).

Older children may use sophisticated strategies to avoid time-out

Third, time-out involving sitting in a chair may be less developmentally appropriate for older children. Pre-teens and adolescents will likely equate sitting on a designated time-out chair or step as "babyish." This adds a punitive

Time-out may be less developmentally appropriate for older children

factor of humiliation to the time-out for older children, which may increase feelings of hostility toward caregivers. Developmentally, older children are better able to benefit from delayed consequences than younger children. Thus, for children in the 7–13-year age range, strategies like restriction of privilege can replace or supplement time-out, which is most beneficial for less mature children who require immediate consequences for optimal learning. Considering these developmental factors, evidence-based behavioral parent training programs often recommend adaptations to the time-out procedure with children over the age of approximately 7 years.

> *Restriction of privilege can replace/supplement time-out*

3.3.1 Managing Time-Out Refusal and Escape

Sometimes, time-out is developmentally appropriate for an older child or adolescent, but for some reason, the child cannot be physically moved to the time-out location. This problem occurs in families of teenagers with developmental disabilities, in families who want to use uniform discipline strategies for all of their children (e.g., siblings ages 4, 6, and 10), and in families where one caregiver may not be able to carry the child to time-out (e.g., physical disabilities, heavy or aggressive child). In these cases, adaptations can be made to manage time-out refusal or escape.

For an older child who refuses to go to time-out, instead of carrying the child to the time-out location, caregivers may offer a restriction of privilege warning for continued noncompliance with time-out. In this situation, a caregiver might say, "If you don't go to time-out, you will lose screen time for the rest of the day." A similar warning can be given to an older child who escapes from the chair after initiating time-out. Although restriction of privilege is technically considered a form of time-out from positive reinforcement itself, most therapists and caregivers do not think of it as time-out. One drawback to the restriction of privilege alternative is that if the child chooses to defy the warning, opting to lose a privilege, the child escapes both the command to sit on the chair and the original command for which noncompliance resulted in time-out. See Chapter 6 for more alternatives.

> *Restriction of privilege if child cannot be moved*

> *Escaping the original command is a drawback to the restriction privilege alternative*

3.3.2 Increasing Buy-In

In addition to physical considerations, modifications to time-out can also target the more sophisticated cognitive abilities and social autonomy of older children. When learning to control their behavior using time-out as a consequence, older children ought to be included in treatment planning. Therapists should consider spending individual time with the older child before working with the family as a whole during each session to increase child buy-in. Older children may respond more cooperatively if they are treated as valuable members of the treatment team. This may mean delineating the benefits of time-out for the child. Namely, the child will no longer be arbitrarily punished without a warning if using the standard therapeutic time-out (outlined in Chapter 8). In this way, the child can be given the power to avoid time-out by obeying the time-out warning if not the original instruction or rule. Decreasing caregivers'

> *Including older children in treatment planning may increase buy-in*

repeated reminding or "nagging" is another benefit of time-out to highlight for older children. Finally, older children appreciate the expectation that time-out helps their parents respond calmly, avoid yelling, refrain from physical discipline, and give predictable consequences.

As an example of a detailed approach for using time-out with older children, the Older Child Protocol for PCIT is described. The Older Child Protocol divides discipline and time-out into three modules (Gibson et al., 2022; McNeil & Hembree-Kigin, 2010). The first module teaches caregivers how to give effective commands followed by specific praise for compliance or a warning and *big ignore* for noncompliance. The big ignore is a very brief, nonexclusionary time-out, which involves the caregiver turning away and ignoring the child's behavior for 45 seconds. The big ignore gives caregivers and older children a chance to get used to the sequence of giving an effective instruction followed by a specific warning and consequence (either praise or big ignore) before introducing a complex standardized therapeutic time-out procedure. Older and more oppositional children may find this gradual introduction to following instructions and accepting consequences less objectionable; therefore, they may be less likely to become aggressive or defiant during discipline. However, the big ignore approach is not a long-term solution as it allows escape from caregiver demands and primarily targets problem behavior driven by negative attention-seeking.

After demonstrating competency with module 1, families progress to module 2. In module 2, the standard time-out procedure replaces the big ignore. An incentive chart is also introduced. Older children can earn a sticker on their incentive chart for each day (or portion of a day) in which they earn zero time-outs or complete any time-outs given. Daily reinforcement (e.g., treat, privilege) may be earned for getting a sticker or a predetermined number of stickers (in the case of breaking the day into portions). In addition, the number of stickers required to earn a larger weekly reward (e.g., bowling, sleepover) is predetermined by the family. Older children should be involved in the selection of motivating rewards as well as the creation of a personalized sticker chart. The incentive chart approach is meant to increase buy-in and facilitate cooperation with sitting in time-out for older children. Warning statements in module 2 are modified to implicate the incentive chart sticker as motivation (e.g., "If you do not walk to the chair, you won't get your sticker." or "You didn't stay on the chair, so you won't get your sticker."; McNeil & Hembree-Kigin, 2010). By using rewards as motivation and not expecting perfection (i.e., stickers may be earned for accepting time-out, even if time-out is earned), module 2 procedures increase the acceptability of time-out for older children. Cognitive strategies and role play are used to help older children practice accepting time-out in sessions.

Lastly, once older children learn to accept time-out consistently, families advance to module 3. Module 3 may not be appropriate for extremely aggressive older children, as it requires the caregiver to suspend privileges until the child accepts the time-out consequence, a procedure that might be dangerous with strong, aggressive children who are prone to attack the caregiver while privileges are suspended. Module 3 typically removes the incentive chart for compliance with rules, instructions, and time-out, as children have already demonstrated significant improvement with these skills. The long-term strategy

---

Time-out warnings decrease repeating, reminding, and nagging

The Older Child Protocol of PCIT

Module 1

Module 2

Module 3

Consider safety with aggressive older children

of time-out with suspension of privilege for time-out refusal or escape is now added. From this point forward, if a child refuses to go to time-out or gets out of time-out without permission, they will lose access to all privileges (e.g., electronics, social engagements, treats, toys, caregiver social attention) until the time-out has been completed. Caregivers are instructed to remove their attention as much as possible and can respond to questions about access to privileges by saying, "I would love for you to have your privileges back. Remember, all you need to do is finish your time-out" (McNeil & Hembree-Kigin, 2010, p. 220). After the time-out, the child is required to complete the original command that resulted in time-out.

Milder and delayed consequences for older children with histories of aggression

For extremely aggressive and defiant older children, the incentive chart should be continued throughout module 3 to sustain cooperation. The suspension of privilege for these children may be modified to a time-delay restriction of specific privileges to which caregivers can more easily control access. Older children who tend to respond impulsively and aggressively to negative consequences may be less likely to "explode" when given a milder, more delayed consequence (e.g., "If you don't go to time-out, there will be no dessert after supper tonight."). Further, caregivers of these children should select privileges that can be controlled with limited risk of physical altercations. For instance, hiding a child's video game remotes in advance is less likely to incite a physical struggle than attempting to block an older child from playing outside. Overall, the Older Child Protocol for PCIT provides a helpful example of how to extend the use of time-out by tailoring it to better accommodate the more mature size, physical abilities, cognitive skills, and social autonomy of older children (Gibson et al., 2022).

3.3.3 Alternative Forms of Time-Out

In some evidence-based programs, caregivers of older children are trained to forgo traditional location-based time-out altogether. Many other behavioral principles (e.g., positive reinforcement, time-in, token systems, compliance training) are still employed. However, time-out is replaced with an alternative. Some popular options include time-based restriction of privilege, loss of points or tokens in a token economy, and task-based restriction of privilege. Although these alternatives are not typically referred to as such, technically, they are all considered to be forms of time-out from positive reinforcement.

Task-based restriction of privilege

While time-based restriction of privilege (e.g., "no friends over for one week") and loss of points in a point system are well-known strategies to many caregivers, task-based restriction of privilege may require some explanation. In task-based restriction of privilege, the older child or adolescent determines how long the consequence will last based on their completion of required task(s). One popular method is called *job card grounding* (Eaves et al., 2005). Using this method, older children or adolescents are "grounded" indefinitely from any privileges that caregivers deem appropriate (e.g., leaving their room, using electronics, going on special outings, eating treats). However, they may regain access to privileges by completing a number of assigned tasks. Caregivers select a variety of developmentally appropriate jobs (e.g., rake leaves, clean out the refrigerator) in advance. Steps are listed in detail on

Job card grounding

Tasks in job card grounding should be developmentally appropriate

separate cards. These jobs should not be tasks already expected of the child, for example, weekly cleaning chores.

When an older child breaks a house rule or refuses to comply with a direct instruction, instead of receiving a time-out, they are grounded, contingent on the completion of a number of job cards assigned. The number of job cards assigned should correlate with the severity of the child's behavior. The older child or adolescent then chooses the card(s) randomly and does not have access to any privileges until the job on the card is completed. Detailed instructions about how to complete the task are included on the card to prevent unnecessary caregiver attention through explaining, prompting, or correcting.

When the older child or adolescent notifies the caregiver that a job is finished, the caregiver checks to see that it has been completed according to the steps detailed. If so, the grounding ends immediately. If not, the older child or adolescent has one more chance to complete it correctly. If again, the job has not been completed to the caregiver's satisfaction, the child may be sent to their room for 1 hour before earning another opportunity to complete the job(s). This limits opportunities for negative attention seeking and motivates diligence. Caregivers can respond to arguing or whining by ignoring this behavior or with the assignment of a second "serving" of job card(s). If a second serving of job cards has been given, continued negative behavior is to be ignored to avoid excessive punishing and escalation. Conversely, if a child accepts consequences calmly, caregivers may reserve the right to randomly remove one of multiple job cards to shape this calm behavior. Adding a reminder about these possibilities immediately before assigning consequences to an older child or adolescent can be useful as well (B. Kuhn, personal communication, February 17, 2021). For example, a caregiver could start by saying, "Remember, your behavior and how well you accept consequences can affect the consequences you earn."

Advantages of task-based restrictions of privilege

Task-based restriction of privilege for older children has advantages. It allows children to determine, to some extent, how long a restriction of privilege lasts. In our clinical experience, oppositional older children and adolescents enjoy feeling some control after receiving a consequence. Working on a task also helps to distract children from the original problem behavior and redirect their energies into a more positive activity. As with traditional time-out, caregivers are relieved of the burden of coming up with a consequence and an appropriate duration for that consequence in the heat of the moment. With task-based restriction of privilege, caregivers and children alike are incentivized to walk away from the conflict and subsequently manage their emotions independently. Last, but not least, lemons are turned into lemonade as the family benefits by having a household task or two completed in the process.

Drawbacks to task-based restriction of privilege

Drawbacks to task-based restriction of privilege should also be presented to families before implementing. Although task-based restriction of privilege relieves caregivers of having to physically move children, they must be able to ensure restriction of access to all implicated desirable activities and objects. A plan for securing items such as remotes, chargers, electric cords, keys, etc. should be discussed with the family in advance. In addition, if a child does not complete the task quickly, caregivers must manage access to these preferred items and activities for extended periods of time. Finally, caregivers must be able to avoid providing reminders, nagging, and criticizing in addition to avoiding children's negative attention seeking bids, after the tasks have been assigned. This, too, should be discussed in advance. Delineating specific preventative strategies (e.g., parent goes to another room, role play) may be helpful.

4

Diversity Issues

Each family's diverse cultural context should inform the use of caregiving practices, and time-out is no exception. In this chapter, we introduce theoretical and evidence-based rationales regarding how a variety of demographic factors such as ethnic, cultural, national group membership, and other socioeconomic factors may interact with time-out implementation. It is important to note that, while some available research sheds light on these issues, members of demographic groups are unique individuals and do not demonstrate all characteristics of each group in a stereotyped manner.

4.1 Ethnic, Racial, and National Considerations

Shared ethnic, racial, and national norms and values are likely to impact views and implementation regarding time-out differently among different cultural groups. Cultural differences in the values of interdependence, respect for authority, demonstrating affection, and providing reinforcement for positive child behavior are commonly cited as influential in the parenting literature. Relatedly, outcomes of disciplinary practices, in general, vary by culture. In a review of cross-cultural literature, it was concluded that discipline practices are more likely to be successful and associated with fewer negative outcomes if children experience them as culturally "normative, fair, and a sign of caring" (Grusec et al., 2017, p. 465). Authors of this review surmised that collectivist cultures view and experience stricter parenting practices less negatively, in part because limiting self-interest and increasing obedience elevates the goals of the larger group (e.g., family, community). Conversely, Westernized cultures tend to view and experience strict discipline more negatively because it is seen as violating values of individual freedom and autonomy.

Views and implementation may differ between cultural groups

How do these multicultural findings about discipline come into play regarding time-out specifically? As with all types of research, experiences of minority cultures are often undervalued (Sue, 2004) and are largely left out of the time-out literature. Time-out was primarily developed by and has been researched mainly on European-American families in the United States. Most studies of time-out acceptability have either focused on majority Caucasian or ethnically European populations (Forcino et al., 2019; Jones et al., 1998; Passini et al., 2014; Rodgers, 1992; Woodfield et al., 2020) or have not reported demographic data on race, ethnicity, or nationality at all (Arndorfer et al., 1999; Blampied & Kahan, 1992; Dadds et al., 1987; Everett et al., 2010; Hobbs et al., 1984; Kazdin, 1980; Singh & Katz, 1985). Consequently, the

Minority cultures are often undervalued and excluded from research

available knowledge in this area must be pieced together, and the results are incomplete.

4.1.1 Minority Groups in the United States

Only a few studies have been conducted on time-out and minority groups in the US. The National Survey of Early Childhood Health (2000) is one of the most informative pieces of research available on the topic. Data revealed that 70% of all caregivers reported using time-out with children between the ages of 19 and 35 months in the United States (Regalado et al., 2004). No significant differences in time-out usage were reported among other ethnic or racial groups, except for Spanish-speaking Hispanic parents, who were less likely than non-Hispanic White parents to use time-out (Regalado et al., 2004). Relatedly, Puerto Rican researchers implementing PCIT tailored to the population received parent feedback that the time-out-focused discipline component was experienced as "too demanding for parents," but treatment overall was ultimately effective and deemed satisfactory by parents (Matos et al., 2006, as cited in Anhalt & Borrego, 2010, p. 367). In one of the only other evaluations of time-out acceptability in minority culture parents, the time-out focused discipline phase of PCIT was considered equally acceptable by Native American and non-Native American families (Anhalt & Borrego, 2010).

Time-out may be viewed as a majority culture, "American" practice

Drawing from the extant research on cultural views, it appears that time-out may be viewed as a majority culture "American" practice. Themes from contemporary research indicate that first generation immigrants to the United States from Korea, for example, were more likely to view time-out as more "American" and corporal punishment as "Korean style" (Kim & Hong, 2007). This study showed that longer periods of residence in the US were associated with greater adherence to "American" standards of parenting. Similarly, a qualitative study of inner-city parents who had immigrated to the US from 27 separate countries reported a belief in strict discipline, including corporal punishment, as a unified theme (McEvoy et al., 2005).

Minority cultural groups may view time-out with distrust

Because time-out can be seen as a White, middle-class, "American" technique, thinking about its use from other cultural perspectives in crucial. Minority cultural groups may view time-out and therapists advocating its use with distrust. Ethnic and racial minority groups have a long history of forced assimilation in the United States. Therefore, majority culture therapists in particular should educate themselves about the sensitive context of "training" caregivers from minority groups in Westernized parenting techniques (Anhalt & Borrego, 2010; Capous et al., 2016; Sue, 2004). Further, using time-out in the context of treatment for mental or behavioral problems may include its own stigma. Various ethnic and racial groups, on average, experience this stigma differently. In response to these issues, McCabe and colleagues (2020) developed a practical personalization approach for tailoring behavioral parent training, including time-out, to enhance the cultural sensitivity of evidence-based parenting techniques for a variety of ethnic groups. Finally, because racial and ethnic minority groups are more likely, on average, to value interdependence and multigenerational family involvement, it is important to evaluate all involved caregivers' views of time-out during therapy (Anhalt &

It is important to evaluate all caregivers' views of time-out during therapy

Borrego, 2010). Clinically, we have experienced barriers to time-out implementation when grandparents in such families express disapproval of parents' use of the time-out procedure. Overall, before implementation, a conversation should be had about how each family member may experience the recommendation of using time-out in relation to cultural values. Based on the available research, and lack thereof, this is especially important for ethnic and racial minority families.

4.1.2   International Views

How do families respond to time-out outside of the United States? Limited research has been conducted assessing the acceptability of time-out outside of the US. For instance, in Switzerland, Passini and colleagues (2014) found that mothers rated time-out as moderately to highly acceptable, preferring it over spanking, yelling, and planned ignoring. Several of the leading behavioral parent training programs which use time-out, like The Incredible Years (Webster-Stratton, 2001), PCIT (Eyberg & Funderburk, 2011), and Triple P (Sanders et al., 2003), have been disseminated widely across the world, and some treatment acceptability data have been collected. For example, Taiwanese researchers implementing PCIT noted that Chinese parents valued respect for authority and typically responded more favorably to the discipline components of treatment, which revolve around time-out, than to the relationship building phase of treatment (Bjørseth et al., 2010).

Responses of families to time-out outside the US

The inclusion of time-out in behavioral parent training is not always adopted. For example, Norwegian therapists have reported viewing time-out as, too "harsh," and ethical and legal concerns about room time-outs in particular have necessitated the use of alternative back-up procedures (Bjørseth et al., 2010). Concerns have been reported in Australia as well. The Australian Association for Infant Mental Health (AAIMHI) fears that children, especially those under the age of 3, will not learn to regulate their feelings while in time-out (AAIMHI, 2016). AAIMHI and a popular attachment-based parenting intervention, Circle of Security, advocate instead for what they call *time-in*. This definition of time-in implies that caregivers offer support, proximity, and guidance during child tantrums instead of overtly discouraging the behavior (AAIMHI, 2016). In an Australian study using a predominantly ethnically Japanese sample, caregivers ranked time-out lower than all other parenting skills taught in the Triple P program regarding perceived usefulness (Matsumoto et al., 2007). Caregivers in the study ranked praise, affection, and talking to children as more useful skills. Of note, the Triple P – Positive Parenting Program originated in Australia.

Time-out may not always be adopted in BPT outside the US

Conflicting views are also evident in New Zealand. Although the Ministry of Health recently endorsed the use of time-out during parent training (Ministry of Health NZ, 2019), acceptability research results have been mixed. On one hand, a community-based sample of educated New Zealanders rated time-out as an acceptable consequence for noncompliance, rating physical discipline as less acceptable and social reprimands and response cost (e.g., restriction of privilege) as more acceptable (Blampied & Kahan, 1992). On the other hand, a qualitative study of therapists in New Zealand reported a unifying theme listing time-out as a barrier to implementing PCIT. Therapists in the study described concerns that time-out was perceived negatively by families, colleagues, and therapists themselves (Woodfield et al., 2020).

4.1.3 Summary

Drawing conclusions about the acceptability of time-out across ethnic, racial, and national groups based on existing research is difficult. It appears that time-out is often interpreted differently within the cultural context. There is some evidence that time-out *can* be an effective intervention if families, therapists, and other stakeholders find it an acceptable practice. Clearly, more research is needed to better understand time-out's global acceptability and the potential need for modifications. Research and implementation conducted by and with minority cultural groups in this effort is crucial (Anhalt & Borrego, 2010; Bjørseth et al., 2010; Blampied & Kahan, 1992; Matsumoto et al., 2007; Woodfield et al., 2020).

4.2 Time-Out in Relation to Other Socioeconomic Factors

Research about time-out in relation to demographic variables is limited

Whereas time-out research and guidelines considering the experiences of racial and ethnic minority groups are rare, our knowledge about time-out in relation to other demographic factors is extremely rare. In general, caregiving practices are influenced by a variety of other cultural variables. Life experiences including poverty, substance abuse, military service, intimate partner violence, trauma, divorce, and incarceration have demonstrated powerful effects on children and their caregivers. In addition, personal variables, such as physical health (e.g., strength, mobility) and abilities (e.g., vision, hearing), developmental functioning (e.g., autism, ADHD, language disorders), and mental health (e.g., mood disorders) greatly impact the ways individuals parent and are parented. Finally, social factors such as gender, religious views, number of adults and children in the home, education, and employment are prominent variables in the larger parenting literature.

While no research was found regarding many of these factors in relation to time-out specifically, a small amount is known about how time-out is experienced based on socioeconomic status (SES). In the following studies, SES was determined by household income and parents' level of education. From 1988–2011, less frequent use of time-out and greater reliance on physical discipline was reported by parents from lower SES groups as compared with those in higher SES groups in the US (Ryan et al., 2016). Still, the popularity and use of time-out appeared to be increasing regardless of income. In large longitudinal samples, Ryan and colleagues found that American mothers across socioeconomic groups reported significant increases in their use of time-out and significant decreases in their use of spanking over the same 25-year period (Ryan et al., 2016). Discipline studies in general have shown that parenting strategies rated as more controlling assertions of power are experienced and viewed less negatively in lower SES contexts around the world (Bugental & Grusec, 2006; Kelley et al., 1992). These authors have theorized that ensuring a child's safety by imposing more control in relatively dangerous low SES environments may be a determinant.

Consideration of cultural context is vital to high quality parenting strategies and interventions as a whole. We hope that this brief review of research and theory regarding the ways in which some unique cultural groups experience time-out will better inform practitioners' work with diverse families. We also wish to highlight the great value that further research in this area would bring. Ensuring equitable access to evidence-based interventions is only possible if the evidence represents all types of families.

Inclusive research is needed to improve equitable access

5

Evidence-Based Programs Including Time-Out

Time-out is used in many treatment programs

Many BPT programs are modeled after Hanf's two-stage program

Time-out is incorporated as a component of almost every evidence-based treatment program for child externalizing behavior problems. One reason for this is that several of the most widely used, well-supported behavioral parent training (BPT) programs were modeled in some way after Constance Hanf's two-stage program, which used time-out (Hanf, 1969). Designed for children 3–7 years of age, Hanf's program focused first on developing positive caregiver–child interactions and on relationship building (the Child's Game) and then calm, consistent discipline strategies (the Parent's Game). Time-out was part of this second phase. Here, we briefly summarize a few of the most widely used evidence-based treatment models for child behavior problems and describe how time-out fits into each. Further resources for parents and caregivers about these programs can be found in Appendix 1.

5.1 The Defiant Children Program

Defiant Children (Barkley, 2013) was developed to improve externalizing behavior problems for children who may also be diagnosed with other psychological disorders (e.g., attention-deficit/hyperactivity disorder [ADHD]; autism spectrum disorder). Its creator, Russel Barkley, has published a variety of books using similar strategies to address problem behavior, particularly geared toward individuals with ADHD (Barkley, 2014). The Defiant Children program is recommended for use with children whose receptive language abilities are equivalent or better than those of a typically developing 24-month-old and is appropriate for children whose developmental level ranges up through that of a typically developing 12-year-old. The program is designed to last for about 10 individual sessions.

10-session program appropriate for ages 2–12 years

Program goals

Defiant Children targets improving parent management of oppositional behavior, increasing caregiver understanding of social causes of defiance, increasing child compliance, and decreasing caregiver stress. After learning about the causes of noncompliance, caregivers learn how to differentially attend to positive behavior by praising it, narrating it, and ignoring minor misbehavior. Caregivers also learn to praise successively longer periods of independent play and compliance to effective instructions. In addition, Barkley's program employs a token economy. Within the token economy, children earn chips or points for engaging in specific positive behavior. Tokens can be exchanged for rewards. Later, children may lose tokens for negative behavior.

Token economy

Another unique component of Defiant Children is the incorporation of a daily school behavior report card. The child's teacher notes progress toward behavioral or academic goals at school and sends the note home each day. In some cases, the token economy may be made contingent on the daily school behavior report.

Because the token economy may be insufficient to manage more challenging defiant or noncompliant behavior, Defiant Children also incorporates the use of time-out. Families choose two behaviors to target with time-out, for example, aggression or noncompliance to a specific instruction. Following the specified behavior, the child is given a warning statement. If the child does not stop the behavior or comply with instruction in 5 seconds, a time-out in a chair is instituted. Each time-out lasts for about 1–2 minutes per year of the child's age. Time-out ends when the child is quiet for a brief period and complies with the original command. Caregivers manage time-out escape or refusal in one of three ways: (1) deducting of points/chips within the token economy, (2) lengthening time-out by 5–10 minutes, or (3) moving the child to a bedroom with entertaining items removed and door locked. After time-out is established as a consequence for the two initially selected types of behavior, time-out can be extended to treat a small number of other problem behaviors. In public, caregivers can have children serve a time-out lasting half as long as time-out at home, near a wall. Alternatively, caregivers can record the infraction in a notebook and have the child complete the time-out upon returning home.

Incorporation of time-out

5.2 Family Interaction Training Program (FIT)

The Family Interaction Training Program (FIT) was developed through a cooperative agreement between the Association of University Centers on Disabilities and the Centers for Disease Control and Prevention in 2018. All materials to administer and complete FIT for both providers and families are available at no cost on the program's website (https://www.aucd.org/template/page.cfm?id=1023). The FIT program can be provided to families by any professional with expertise in training, teaching, clinical work, or therapy geared toward parents. FIT combines a variety of some of the most effective parenting strategies gleaned from other evidence-based models to guide caregivers in managing disruptive behavior in young children. FIT was derived from The Incredible Years (Webster-Stratton & Reid, 2017), parent–child interaction therapy (PCIT; Eyberg & Funderburk, 2011), Positive Parenting Program (Triple P; Sanders et al., 2003), and the New Forest Parenting Programme (Thompson et al., 2009).

FIT materials for providers and families are available online at no cost

The goal of the FIT project is to create affordable, public access to evidence-based treatment for families and providers who may not otherwise have access. Many of the other evidence-based models in this chapter require providers to obtain costly training certifications, advanced behavioral degrees, and access to copyrighted materials. In addition, treatment through other models often necessitates weekly, in-person therapy attendance, which creates its own barriers (e.g., cost, time, travel, childcare) for families. Research is

Program goals

currently being conducted on the dissemination, implementation, and effectiveness of the FIT model.

The FIT program instructs providers in the methods of facilitating BPT for families. Providers can access free training via the FIT website (https://www.aucd.org/template/news.cfm?news_id=12130&id=17). The website offers a trainer's manual, video lessons for trainers, and caregiver handouts, quizzes, worksheets, videos, and homework materials. Providers learn to lead families through BPT content organized into three modules: (1) strengthening the parent–child relationship; (2) structuring the environment to prevent misbehavior; and (3) effective strategies for addressing misbehavior. Typical family sessions include reviewing homework, viewing new content videos, discussing content, role playing, completing quizzes or worksheets, and developing behavior plans. Child attendance is not required. The entire program is structured to be completed in 14 sessions or fewer.

Lesson 12 in module 3 of the FIT Program is entirely devoted to training caregivers to use time-out. The FIT Program advocates a 2–3 minute time-out in a chair or quiet space. Time-out is administered for noncompliance to instruction. Children are allowed 3–5 seconds to comply after the instruction and after 1 warning statement before being sent to time-out. Children are required to be quiet for a few seconds at the end of time-out and to comply with the original instruction. "Automatic time-outs" can also be used for pre-selected unacceptable behavior (e.g., aggression) in the FIT program. If children refuse to go to time-out, the program instructs caregivers in two alternatives: (1) remove all toys and people from the child's current environment, effectively creating an in-place time-out; or (2) offer a different consequence, such as restriction of privilege. If a child escapes or engages in unsafe behavior during time-out, FIT recommends stopping the unsafe behavior or putting the child back repeatedly while providing as little attention as possible. The clock for time-out starts over each time a caregiver intervenes.

The FIT program advocates for the importance of time-in and positive attention throughout its lessons. Caregivers are encouraged to save long explanations about the misbehavior that warranted time-out for another time. This helps parents focus instead on creating positive caregiver–child interactions immediately following time-out. Providers and caregivers role-play time-out in session before implementing the procedure at home. Caregivers are encouraged to demonstrate time-out with a doll for their child before using time-out for the first time.

5.3 The Helping the Noncompliant Child Program

Helping the Noncompliant Child (HNC; McMahon & Forehand, 2003) is an evidence-based treatment program for child behavior problems, which focuses on improving child compliance as the central component. Appropriate for children ages 3–8 years, HNC sessions involve both the caregiver and child in every session. The authors also wrote a popular press version of this program as a parent resource (Forehand & Long, 2010). As a Hanf-derived program, treatment involves two phases. First, in the differential attention phase, caregivers practice providing social attention for desirable child behavior, ignoring minor undesirable behavior, and decreasing their own directive verbal behavior. After caregivers demonstrate proficiency in the differential attention phase skills, the compliance training phase begins. In this phase, caregivers learn the *clear instructions sequence*, which involves delivering clear, concise instructions and offering positive attention for compliance or time-out for noncompliance. Later in the second phase, standing rules are put in place, and skills are extended to situations outside of the home. Treatment involves 60–90-minute family sessions, 1–2 times per week for approximately 8-10 sessions (McMahon & Forehand, 2003). **Treatment phases**

Within HNC, the time-out procedure is designed as follows. Following delivery of a clear instruction from a caregiver, a child is given 5 seconds in which to comply. If no effort toward compliance is made, the caregiver issues a warning statement. Following noncompliance to the warning statement, the caregiver places the child in the time-out chair for 3 minutes. The child must remain quiet for 15 seconds at the end of the 3-minute period in order to be released from the chair. Compliance with the original command is then required. During time-out, if the child removes their bottom from the chair for one second or more, the caregiver may use one of three back-up procedures: (1) require a second 3-minute chair time-out; (2) move the child to a back-up room; or (3) remove a privilege or issue some other response cost (for older children). Refusal to go to time-out in the first place is also handled using one of these three options. **Incorporation of time-out**

5.4 The Incredible Years Program

The Incredible Years (IY; Webster-Stratton & Reid, 2017) is an interconnected family of evidence-based interventions which may be used to help teachers, caregivers, and children increase social competence and reduce behavior problems. The program was originally developed to prevent and treat conduct problems in children ages 3–8 years. Currently, facets of programming promote behavioral health in children from 0–12 years of age. **Program goals**

Appropriate for ages 0–12

Within the IY programs, time-out is described as an opportunity for children to calm down, regulate emotions, and reflect on better problem-solving solutions, rather than a punishment. Caregivers and teachers also learn to use this time as a break to regulate themselves and to model better responding to emotional upsets. Prior to implementing time-out, therapists and caregivers discuss and use puppets to introduce the importance of calming down during emotional upsets. IY uses time-out to reduce aggression, destructive behavior, and noncompliance (The Incredible Years, 2013; Webster-Stratton, 2001).

Similar to the procedure used in HNC, noncompliance to a command and warning statement is followed by the directive, "Go to time out." Time-out, as taught in the IY programs, lasts for 1 minute per year of child age with an upper limit of 5 minutes (Havighurst et al., 2013). Refusal to go to the chair prompts a choice-giving statement for use with younger children (e.g., "You can walk to time out like a big boy/girl or I will take you there."). Older children who refuse to go to time-out receive an additional minute of time-out **Incorporation of time-out** up to 9 minutes, followed by restriction of privilege, for continued refusal. A back-up room is used for escape (i.e., leaving time-out without permission). Compliance with the original instruction is required to return to play. Time-out is followed by emphasis on reaffirming the positive relationship between caregiver and child (e.g., warm touches, positive affirmations).

5.5 Parent–Child Interaction Therapy (PCIT)

Program goal: Treating disruptive behavior problems

Parent–child interaction therapy (PCIT; Eyberg & Funderburk, 2011; McNeil & Hembree-Kigin, 2010) is an evidence-based BPT approach originally developed to treat disruptive behavior problems. PCIT is appropriate for children ages 2–7 years. During about 12–20, 1-hour weekly sessions, caregivers learn and practice skills with their child with bug-in-the-ear coaching from a therapist. Treatment unfolds in two phases. In the child-directed interaction phase, caregivers learn positive reinforcement skills (i.e., praise, reflect, imitate, describe, enjoy [PRIDE]). These are to be practiced daily during 5 minutes of one-on-one child-led play at home. Next, during the parent-directed interaction phase, caregivers practice calm, consistent discipline strategies for noncompliance. PCIT is competency-based, meaning that families' progression through treatment is guided by caregivers' attainment of competency goals (e.g., 10 praises, reflections, and descriptions in 5 minutes, 75% correct follow-through with discipline skills).

12–20-session program in 2 phases and appropriate for ages 2–7

Incorporation of time-out

Within the parent-directed interaction phase of treatment, time-out is used as a consequence for noncompliance. Children are given one warning before the time-out sequence is initiated. Time-out occurs in a chair and lasts for 3 minutes plus 5 seconds of silence. Following this period, the child must comply with the original instruction to end time-out. Caregivers are coached through the scripted steps of time-out with their child in clinic before practicing at home. Immediately following all time-outs, caregivers are encouraged to provide ample positive reinforcement using the PRIDE skills. This highlights the differential reinforcement of desirable behavior as compared with noncompliance. More details on the time-out procedure used in PCIT are provided in Chapter 8.

5.6 The Kazdin Method (Formerly Parent Management Training)

Program goal: Developing desirable behavior

The Kazdin method, formerly known as Parent Management Training (PMT; Kazdin, 2005, 2008), is an evidence-based BPT program. PMT was originally developed to address conduct problems (e.g., aggression, property destruction). The Kazdin Method now aims to develop desirable behavior and values. The Kazdin method is designed for families of children ages 2–15 years. Within 5–10, 1-hour weekly therapy sessions, caregivers learn basic behavior management skills such as shaping, modeling, prompting, fading, reinforcement, punishment, and extinction (Kazdin, 2008). Children do not attend

5–10-session program for caregivers of children aged 2–15

sessions, but therapists work with caregivers using modeling, rehearsal, and role play. Recently, the Kazdin method has been developed into an online course entitled, *Everyday Parenting: The ABCs of Childrearing*. Caregivers can audit the course for free through Coursera, and it is available with subtitles in at least six languages (https://www.coursera.org/learn/everyday-parenting).

As a whole, the Kazdin method does not emphasize punishment. In fact, Kazdin cautions against the overuse of punishment, touting its immediate risks, such as inciting aggression, escalation, and tantrums. As part of a larger treatment package underscoring the importance of time-in, praise, and positive opposites, Kazdin explicitly instructs caregivers about how to conduct time-out. The Kazdin method advocates a time-out lasting between 1 and 10 minutes, preferably between 2 and 5 minutes. The location for time-out is not specific, and families can choose an area where the child does not have access to reinforcing activities or attention. This may even mean simply discontinuing participation in current activities while remaining in the original environment. Kazdin discourages physical contact between caregivers and children during time-out (e.g., guiding, carrying the child), citing increased risk of aggression, force, and escalation. The Kazdin method also encourages caregivers to determine a back-up consequence for not accepting time-out; one option is a restriction of privilege. Back-ups are used after the provision of a warning or choice regarding refusal to go to time-out. Finally, all of these components must be agreed upon in advance. Kazdin strongly encourages caregivers and their children to be clear about expectations and to practice the time-out procedure before implementing (Kazdin, 2008).

Incorporation of time-out

5.7 Triple P – Positive Parenting Program

Triple P – Positive Parenting Program (PPP; Sanders et al., 2003) is an evidence-based family of prevention and intervention programs. Its goals are to target children's developmental, emotional, and behavioral health through parent education and training. Triple P is unique in that it is multi-tiered, ranging from population-based prevention (e.g., national media campaigns) to intensive therapy (Sanders, 1999). As with the other programs described here, Triple P strikes a balance of imparting positive parenting skills to increase positive behavior (e.g., social skills, problem solving) and teaching child behavior management techniques (e.g., differential attention, time-out). Triple P can be administered in as few as 1–2 sessions in a primary care office or as many as 10, 2-hour group therapy sessions over the course of 8 weeks, supplemented with individual telephone check-ins. Triple P has now been adapted into an online parenting course, *Triple P Online*, consisting of 8, 30–60-minute modules (https://www.triplep-parenting.com/us/triple-p/).

Program goals

1–10-session program for caregivers of children aged 2–10 years

Triple P recommends time-out as an appropriate intervention for children ages 2–10 years. The program advocates using time-out for aggression. More specifically, time-out can be used when a child does not comply with a caregiver's directive to stop aggressive behavior and engage in a more positive replacement behavior. Following 5 seconds of noncompliance, Triple P recommends moving the child to a safe but boring area. During a Triple P

Incorporation of time-out

time-out, the child must remain quiet for a designated period of time: 1 minute for 2-year-olds and up to 5 minutes for older children. The rule about being quiet is restated for the child at the start of the time-out period. Refusal to go to time-out is handled by carrying the child. For escape, Triple P recommends holding the door to the time-out area closed or repeatedly taking the child back to the area with as little interaction as possible. Following time-out, caregivers are discouraged from discussing or lecturing about the child's negative behavior. Caregivers are encouraged to provide positive reinforcement for more prosocial behavior. As an alternative to its traditional time-out, Triple P also uses a version called quiet time (Sanders, 2008). During quiet time, the child is allowed to remain in the original environment where misbehavior occurred, while the caregiver engages in planned ignoring.

5.8 Summer Treatment Program

Program goals: Management of ADHD and other problem behavior 6–9 week program appropriate for ages 5–16

The Children's Summer Treatment Program (STP; Pelham et al., 2019) is a 6- to 9-week, evidence-based day camp style program originally developed for the treatment of ADHD. Children ages 5–16 participate within groups of 12–15 same-aged peers. Camp staff facilitate behaviorally focused contingency management throughout the day, which centers on a token economy, while campers engage in structured activities (Fabiano et al., 2014). Children earn points for exhibiting desirable behavior (e.g., following directions) and lose points for demonstrating less desirable behavior (e.g., interrupting). Points are communicated through a daily report card shared with caregivers at home. Points can be cashed in for privileges and rewards at camp or at home. Other components to the Summer Treatment Program include a weekly BPT group, 2 hours of daily academic work, social skills training, and medication evaluations.

Token economy

Incorporation of time-out

In addition to its token economy, the Summer Treatment Program uses time-out to manage behavior. Time-out is implemented as a consequence for clearly defined egregious behavior like physical aggression or ongoing noncompliance (Fabiano et al., 2014). Time-out duration is typically 10–30 minutes, with the longer durations being used for older children. Children may earn a 50% reduction in time-out duration as a reward for positive behavior related to accepting time-out. To make time-in more reinforcing, a variety of strategies are employed. Camp staff interact with children enthusiastically, offer enjoyable activities (e.g., swimming, art), praise often, share children's successes with caregivers, recognize good behavior publicly, and facilitate positive social interactions with others. Taken together, the approaches used in the Summer Treatment Program have demonstrated a strong evidence base for the management of ADHD and other problem behavior (Pelham et al., 1998).

5.9 Parent Management Training – Oregon/ Generation PMT–O

Parent Management Training – Oregon (PMT-O; Forgatch & Patterson, 2010; Patterson, 2005) is a group of manualized, evidence-based treatments aimed at decreasing antisocial behavior in children and teens. The model operates under the assumption that the identified child's aggressive or inappropriate behavior can be modified by changes in the social environments or how others respond (Reid et al., 2002). Drawing heavily on Patterson's coercive process (Patterson, 1979), PMT–O aims to interrupt cycles of escalation. In these cycles, family members have learned to become increasingly aggressive to escape others' demands or to get their own demands met. The five main treatment areas in PMT–O are skill encouragement, limit setting, parental monitoring, problem solving, and positive involvement. Treatment occurs in a family-based or group format. Group therapy occurs over about 14, 90-minute sessions, while family therapy lasts for 25–30, 1-hour sessions (Forgatch & Gewirtz, 2017).

Program goal: Management of antisocial beheavior

14 group or 25–30 family therapy sessions

Within the core component of limit setting, caregivers are taught to use time-out as a consequence for noncompliance, aggression, inappropriate language, or conflict among siblings. Time-out duration is 5 minutes with additional minutes (up to 10) for noncompliance with time-out. If, after adding time up to 10 minutes, the child still refuses time-out, a 15–30 minute removal of privilege is used as a back-up. However, younger children can be carried to time-out as a back-up. Caregivers are trained in time-out procedures and must demonstrate proficiency before using time-out outside of session. Proficiency is required in both positive reinforcement skills (i.e., at least a 5:1 ratio to negative parenting skills) and role play of discipline strategies. Proficiency includes delivering time-out immediately, calmly, and consistently, while keeping physical distance and limiting unnecessary verbalizations (Forgatch & Patterson, 2010).

Incorporation of time-out

5.10 Summary

Time-out is a popular component of many empirically supported BPT models. While it is certainly not the only contributing factor, time-out is a pillar of effective limit setting and discipline training within these programs. Time-out specifications vary slightly from model to model. However, emphasis on time-out delivery in the context of positive caregiver–child relationships and shaping positive alternatives to problem behavior are consistent across the board. See Box 1 for common time-out components across many evidence-based programs.

Time-out is an effective component within BPT training programs

Box 1
Common Time-Out Components Across Many Evidence-Based Programs

Effective commands

Warning statements

Relatively short time-out length

Increased positive reinforcement in the environment at other times to distinguish from decreased reinforcement in time-out environment

Back-up consequences for escape from time-out (e.g., carrying young children to back-up room, restricting privileges for older children)

Requirement for child to comply with original command after time-out

Increased positive interaction with the child immediately following time-out

6

Parameters of Time-Out

Before beginning our overview of commonly delineated parameters of time-out, we would first like to highlight a crucial factor related to time-out: time-in. As time-out is more fully understood as time out from positive reinforcement, its effectiveness is enhanced by increasing the quality and amount of positive reinforcement available in the child's environment. Therefore, to ensure the effectiveness of time-out, time-in should involve high levels of reinforcement (e.g., positive caregiver interaction, stimulating activities, and access to other reinforcers; Hernstein, 1955; Solnick et al., 1977). Experts have noted that this is one of the most vital components of time-out efficacy (Shriver & Allen, 1996). Partially for this reason, many evidence-based treatments that teach time-out also prescribe intentional practices aimed at enhancing the caregiver–child relationship. Parent–child interaction therapy trains and coaches caregivers to engage in positive parenting skills for 5 minutes each day with their children. These habits are intended to "spill out" to other times of day, wherein the caregiver continues to improve the reinforcing nature of caregiver–child interactions. Without this basic component of quality time-in, time-out would be far less effective.

Several reviews have been published covering research related to the core components of time-out (Brantner & Doherty, 1983; Corralejo, Jensen, Greathouse, & Ward, 2018; Everett et al., 2010; Harris, 1985; Hobbs & Forehand, 1977; MacDonough & Forehand, 1973; Turner & Watson, 1999). Originally, MacDonough and Forehand (1973) examined eight such components: (1) **verbalized reason** (presence vs. absence); (2) **warning** (presence vs. absence); (3) **administration** (instructional vs. physical); (4) **location** (isolated vs. nonisolated); (5) **duration** (short vs. long); (6) **stimulus** (signaled vs. nonsignaled); (7) **schedule** (continuous vs. intermittent); and (8) **release** (contingent vs. noncontingent). Most recently, Corralejo and colleagues (2018) revisited this list, updating their review to include more recent research. Overall, relatively little empirical evidence exists informing practitioners and parents about the comparative efficacy of each specific parameter of time-out.

Descriptions and summaries of the available evidence behind each parameter are provided below. Discussion of the **stimulus** parameter has been omitted from our review as no research on the comparative effects of different time-out stimuli has been conducted. However, we have included an additional parameter, **escape** from time-out, in our review.

> Time-in enhances the effectiveness of time-out
>
> Time-in should involve high levels of positive reinforcement
>
> Eight core components of time-out

6.1 Verbalized Reason

A simple and short explanation of why time-out is warranted

In this context, a verbalized reason is a simple statement of explanation, given to a child, about what behavior occurred to warrant a time-out. "You hurt your brother, so you have to go to time-out" is an example. Verbalized reasons in the three studies available on this topic were provided or described as occurring before the child was directed to time-out (Alevizos & Alevizos; 1975; Gardner et al., 1976; Rodgers, 1992). In theory, specifying the reason for time-out may help a child learn more quickly or generalize to similar behavior (e.g., labeling "hurting" could help the child generalize the consequence for hitting to other types of hurting behavior). Although this topic has received little research attention, the two available studies which directly investigated this parameter found no difference in effectiveness between time-outs with and without verbalized reasons given immediately prior (Alevizos & Alevizos; 1975; Gardner et al., 1976). Though time-out alone can be effective at reducing contingent problem behavior, Rodgers (1992) showed that childcare staff preferred giving a verbalized reason when administering time-out. In contrast, long explanations to a child while being placed in time-out can decrease the effectiveness of time-out by acting as a reinforcer (i.e., attention; Wolf et al., 1964). Further research examining other potential outcomes of using verbalized reasons, such as generalization to other behavior problems, prosocial reasoning, or caregiver–child relationship quality, would be helpful in informing caregivers and practitioners on this topic.

Long explanations may decrease effectiveness

Take-away point: The few studies available in this area suggest that simple verbalized reasons given prior to time-out do not impact effectiveness, although, verbalized reasons may increase social validity and acceptability of the time-out procedure for caregivers.

6.2 Warning

A time-out warning is a prompt which indicates that a time-out will follow if the child does not behave as directed. Some evidence-based treatments recommend using a verbal warning phrased in an "If ..., then" statement; for example, "If you don't ..., you will have to sit in time-out." Theoretically, warnings have three purposes: First, warnings give the child an opportunity to hear the instruction a second time in case they did not hear it or were not paying attention initially. By explicitly restating the original instruction *within* the warning, caregivers can be more confident that any subsequent noncompliance is intentional. Second, a warning serves as a discriminative stimulus. Throughout a typical day, caregivers issue many instructions, not all of which are intended to result in a time-out for noncompliance. By using a warning statement, caregivers can clearly signal which instructions must be obeyed immediately. Third, warning statements allow the child (and caregiver) to avoid time-out. In alignment with the goal of helping children develop self-control, warning statements prompt children to attend to their behavior to avoid negative consequences. Warnings also make salient for children the presence of choice,

Purposes of time-out warning

allowing them to experience more control in the caregiver–child relationship. In other words, giving a warning allows children to decide for themselves whether or not they go to time-out.

Despite theoretical arguments supporting the use of warnings, only four studies have provided empirical evidence about whether warned or unwarned time-outs produce different outcomes. The results are complicated. Roberts (1982) demonstrated that the presence of a warning made no difference in the efficacy of time-out on child compliance. In contrast, Jones et al. (1992) found that time-outs preceded by a prompt (e.g., "don't hit") and then a time-out warning actually increased problem behavior as opposed to unwarned time-outs, which decreased problem behavior. These authors proposed that these two verbalizations may have functioned to reinforce problem behavior by providing attention. Time-out procedures incorporating a single preceding warning, however, have been shown to necessitate fewer time-outs than procedures without warnings (Roberts, 1982; Velasquez et al., 2016). Conversely, when comparing unwarned time-outs with time-outs preceded by three warnings in a classroom setting, Twyman and colleagues (1994) found that, while roughly equal numbers of time-outs were required in both conditions, unwarned time-outs were associated with better compliance. Finally, Velasquez and colleagues (2016) showed decreasing compliance over time with warned time-outs vs. unwarned time-outs for the majority of subjects.

Take-away point: Both time-outs with and without warnings can be effective at improving compliance, but single warnings may necessitate fewer time-outs. Time-out procedures including repeated warnings may be less effective than those with one or no warnings.

6.3 Administration

As conceptualized by MacDonough and Forehand (1973), administration refers to the method by which caregivers implement time-out; this is usually through physical or instructional means. In other words, children can be physically carried or guided to a time-out environment or motivated to move themselves through caregiver instruction. In some cases, initiating time-out through verbal instruction may be more feasible, especially when physical limitations (e.g., child who is heavy or escapes, incapacitated caregiver) or ethical/legal limitations (e.g., staff prohibited from lifting children, history of physical abuse) make physical guidance inappropriate. On the other hand, physical guidance may be preferred to verbal administration when instruction alone is ineffective. For example, some children cannot yet understand instructions or choose not to comply with them.

Administration is the method of implementation

Unfortunately, only one study has specifically compared physically guided and verbal time-out administrations. Donaldson and colleagues (2013) showed that children were more likely to obey instructions to go to time-out independently when offered a reduction in duration of time-out for doing so. Children were less likely to require physical guidance for time-out initiation when offered the chance to reduce time-out length from 4 minutes to 1 minute than without this option. Overall, time-out was equally effective at reducing problem behavior in both conditions.

Take-away point: More research is needed to inform the most effective method for time-out initiation. However, there are no data to suggest that one method, verbal or physical, is superior to the other.

6.4 Location/Type

The location or arrangement of the environment in which time-out is served varies across research studies, evidence-based programs, and real-world settings. Brantner and Doherty (1983) described three types of time-outs, differentiated by location or access to reinforcement. We review each of the three categories, organized from most to least restrictive. To illustrate, an example which targets problem behavior at school is incorporated. In the illustration, the student, Mia, rocks in her chair, making disruptive squeaking noises in the classroom.

6.4.1 Isolation Time-Outs

Isolation from a reinforcing environment

First, isolation time-outs involve isolating the child from a reinforcing environment. This can be done by removing the child from the immediate environment, often to the child's bedroom at home or another back-up room where the child is alone. In our example, Mia's rocking behavior is reinforced by other children laughing (i.e., attention) and the teacher pausing their lesson (i.e., escape). To isolate the child from these sources of reinforcement, she could be sent to the school office for the rest of the class period to do her lesson there. Isolation time-outs require adequate space and supervision. In most cases, they should not be used for more than a few minutes. While highly effective at isolating children from reinforcement, isolation time-outs should be carefully considered from ethical and legal standpoints before implementing.

Ethical and legal standpoints must be considered before implementing

6.4.2 Exclusionary Time-Outs

Separating from the source(s) of reinforcement

Second, exclusionary time-outs separate the child from the source(s) of reinforcement but do not completely isolate the child. In our example, Mia may be asked to sit on the carpet, away from the rest of the students for the rest of the lesson. Therefore, she would be separated from the other children's attention and prevented from interrupting the lesson by rocking her chair, but she would not be completely isolated from the original environment. Exclusionary time-outs may be a feasible option for teachers and caregivers who must supervise multiple children at once. Home and school environments frequently have designated areas such as a time-out chair, mat, or stair-step in the main living area or classroom for this purpose. While in this designated area, children may either be prevented from observing the original activity or be allowed to

A feasible option when multiple children are present

view it (i.e., contingent observation). In some cases, preventing observation may ensure minimal reinforcement during time-out (e.g., not being allowed to watch the television). In others, being allowed to watch the original activity highlights reinforcement which the child cannot currently access (e.g., observing other children enjoying a snack or playing a game).

6.4.3 Nonexclusionary Time-Outs

Third, nonexclusionary time-outs allow the child to remain in place while receiving time-out from specified reinforcement (e.g., attention). Nonexclusionary time-outs can be further divided into three categories: contingent observation, removal of stimulus conditions, and ignoring (Turner & Watson, 1999). In **contingent observation**, sometimes referred to as "sit and watch" in classroom settings, children must observe other children engaging in a given activity without participating themselves. The goal is for the child to observe others being reinforced for positive behavior. After time-out, the child should be reinforced immediately upon engaging in appropriate behavior. With **removal of stimulus conditions**, access to reinforcers is removed during time-out. This may be toys, materials, treats, or the opportunity to earn rewards or points. Several parenting interventions teach caregivers to put toys in time-out by removing them from the child's environment for a short period of time. More detail on this procedure is provided in Chapter 8 under discussion of the swoop and go procedure. It is recommended that access to reinforcers only be returned following appropriate behavior (Turner & Watson, 1999). Finally, **ignoring** involves the removal of social attention. This may implicate caregivers, peers, siblings, and others in the child's immediate environment. During discrete trial training within an applied behavior analysis approach, time-out from social attention may be used as a consequence for a child's incorrect responding. Here, a clinician may turn their face and body away from the child for a few seconds, remaining quiet, to discourage incorrect responding. In our classroom example, ignoring would be accomplished if Mia's teacher instructed the other students not to respond to Mia, and the teacher refrained from responding as well, for the rest of the lesson. The teacher would also continue teaching without pausing in response to Mia's rocking. In this way, Mia would experience time-out from avoidance of the lesson *and* other students' attention without being excluded from the original environment. For removal of stimulus conditions, the teacher could remove Mia's chair, desk, and even schoolwork materials for a short period, having Mia sit on the floor. She could also suspend the chance to earn points on the classroom reinforcement system for Mia during time-out. Lastly, to administer a contingent observation time-out, Mia could be excluded from participating in the lesson (e.g., being called upon, participating in group work) while observing her peers participate. The teacher would focus on providing lots of attention and reinforcement of other students' appropriate behavior during Mia's time-out (e.g., "Thank you for sitting quietly in your chair, Abdul.").

> Time-out from a specific reinforcer but remaining in place

Five studies have explicitly compared the effectiveness of location or type of time-out on effectiveness at reducing target behavior. Three of these studies found similar effectiveness for isolation time-outs (i.e., removal of child from classroom or removal of mother and toys from room) and nonexclusionary time-outs (e.g., removal of social attention; Forehand et al., 1976; Miles & Cuvo, 1980; Scarboro & Forehand, 1975). Notably, quicker behavior change occurred with isolation time-outs in the study involving removal of mother and toys from the room vs. removal of mothers' social attention only (Scarboro & Forehand, 1975). In addition, Forehand and colleagues (1976) showed greater lasting effects for isolation time-outs than nonexclusionary time-outs (e.g., ignoring). Conversely, Rolider and Van Houten (1985) demonstrated that nonexclusionary time-out was more effective than isolation time-out at decreasing self-stimulatory behavior. In this study, nonexclusionary time-out meant physically blocking the subject from engaging in the self-stimulatory behavior. Blocking was not possible in the isolation time-out condition.

Other researchers have specifically compared exclusionary and nonexclusionary time-outs. Kazdin (1980) showed that college students found the *idea* of nonexclusionary time-outs for children to be more acceptable than exclusionary time-outs. In practice, Mace and Heller (1990) found equivalent reductions in disruptive behavior with exclusionary (i.e., sit in the corner) and nonexclusionary (i.e., move chair back from table) time-outs. When target behavior is maintained by automatic reinforcement (i.e., self-stimulation), however, nonexclusionary time-out was superior to exclusionary time-out (Rolider & Van Houten, 1985).

Take-away point: Given the lack of strong evidence that more restrictive locations or types of time-out are more effective, we recommend using the least restrictive option in which time-out from reinforcement can be reliably carried out. Removal from the original environment alone may be less effective for decreasing self-stimulatory behavior as compared with other types of target behavior.

6.5 Duration

What does the literature say about how long a time-out should last to be effective? The answer is complicated, but the focus of the relative time-out duration research can be organized into three categories: (1) brief time-outs, (2) time-outs lasting longer than 15 minutes, and (3) contrast or sequencing effects.

6.5.1 Brief Time-Outs

Research supports brief time-outs

Given that brief time-outs are more acceptable in most contexts because of ethical and time considerations, it would be convenient if brief time-outs were effective. Luckily, research supports this to a large degree. In their study of young, neurodiverse children (i.e., those with ADHD, developmental delays, brain injuries), Corralejo and colleagues (2018) found 1-minute time-outs to be effective at reducing sibling aggression, and there was no need to implement planned extensions of time-out up to 10 minutes. Also lending support to shorter durations, McGuffin (1991) discovered no differences in effectiveness among 5-, 15-, and 20-minute time-outs. Similarly, Pendergrass (1971) found 5- and 20-minute time-outs to be equally effective. Lending further support, 5-, 10-, and 15-minute time-outs were equally effective at reducing problem behavior in children with ADHD at a Summer Treatment Program (Fabiano et al., 2004). However, for 25% of children in the study for whom shorter time-outs were less effective, longer or escalating time-outs (e.g., time was added for negative behavior during time-out) were more effective.

When comparing very brief time-outs (fewer than 5 minutes), some research shows a lower limit of duration for effectiveness. Hobbs and colleagues (1978) showed that 4-minute time-outs were more effective than 10-second and 1-minute time-outs for a group of 4–6-year-olds. Likewise, McGuffin (1991) found that 1-minute time-outs were less effective than 5-minute time-outs for reducing aggression in children with conduct problems. In contrast, Kapalka & Bryk (2007) found no differences in effectiveness among time-out durations of 2 minutes, 4 minutes, 1 minute per year of age, and 2 minutes per year of age for young boys with ADHD. Similarly, James (1976) found that 1-, 5-, 10-, and 30-second time-outs were equally effective at decreasing stuttering in adults.

Differential effectiveness among 5–20-minute time-out durations

6.5.2 Longer Time-Outs

The majority of popular parenting practices and empirically supported parent training programs alike advocate for relatively brief time-outs for child behavior management (e.g., 3–5 minutes, 1 minute for each year of age). Research investigating longer time-outs (i.e., greater than 15 minutes) comes mainly from institutional settings in the 1970 and 1980s. When comparing the effectiveness of 15- and 30-minute time-outs at reducing problem behavior in individuals with intellectual disabilities, White and colleagues (1972) found no significant differences between the two, regardless of sequencing. Similarly, Benjamin and colleagues (1983) showed no differences in the effectiveness of 15-, 30-, 45-, 60-, and 90-minute time-outs for reducing assaultive behavior, regardless of sequence. Interestingly, the length of time it took individuals to settle once put in time-out was positively correlated with the length of the time-out (i.e., longer time-out, longer to settle; Benjamin et al., 1983). In a single case design, Freeman and colleagues (1976) found a 15-minute time-out to be more effective than both a 1-hour and 3-minute time-out, although the child fell asleep during the 1-hour time-out at the 15-minute mark. Each of these studies support the use of time-outs no longer than 15 minutes.

Studies support the use of time-outs no longer than 15 minutes

6.5.3 Contrast or Sequencing Effects

Results of a few time-out duration studies have highlighted the potential for contrast or sequencing effects. Of these, two studies have shown sequencing effects. More specifically, shorter time-outs can be effective, but if they are employed *after* an individual has been exposed to longer time-outs, shorter

Shorter time-outs less effective after exposure to longer time-outs

time-outs may be less effective. For example, for institutionalized individuals with intellectual disabilities, 1-, 15-, and 30-minute time-outs had comparable effectiveness at reducing problem behavior *except* when 1-minute time-outs were used *after* the individual had already experienced one of the longer time-outs (White et al., 1972). Similarly, Kendall and colleagues (1975) demonstrated that 5-minute time-outs reduced problem behavior in delinquent adolescents, but the effect was reduced when individuals had already been exposed to a 30-minute time-out condition. Relatedly, Burchard and Barrera (1972) found that 5-minute time-outs were less effective when contrasted with more severe treatment conditions (i.e., 30-minute time-outs, 30-token response cost, and 5-minute time-out plus 5-token response cost). Theoretically, findings from these three studies have been attributed to contrast effects. To complicate the theory, though, this conclusion directly opposes findings described in the previous section which revealed no contrast or sequencing effects among time-outs exclusively lasting 15 minutes or longer (Benjamin et al., 1983; White et al., 1972).

Take-away point: Much research supports the effectiveness of relatively brief time-outs (i.e., 5 minutes or fewer). There is little if any effectiveness to be gained by increasing time-out duration beyond 15 minutes and in some cases beyond 5 minutes. There is no evidence supporting a "magic formula" to determine the shortest effective duration among those times shorter than 5 minutes as results have varied by population, setting, and problem behavior. Brief time-outs (shorter than 15 minutes) may be less effective if they follow or contrast with a child's exposure to a longer or more severe consequence.

6.6 Schedule

Schedule refers to how often or how consistently time-out is implemented

In behavioral science, schedule refers to the rate or frequency with which stimuli (e.g., reinforcers, punishers) are applied in relation to target behavior. When applied to time-out, schedule refers to how often or how consistently time-out is implemented following a target behavior. In behavioral research in general, more consistent application of punishment produces the greatest reductions in target responding (Azrin et al., 1963). Therefore, it would be expected that using a time-out consistently for each instance of a child's behavior that caregivers wish to reduce (e.g., hitting siblings) would reduce that behavior more effectively than using time-out less consistently (e.g., after the child hits a few times).

Consistent time-outs are more effective

There is time-out research to back up this hypothesis. Pendergrass (1971) and Calhoun and Matherne (1975) showed that more consistent use of time-out reduced children's aggressive behavior better than less consistent use (e.g., time-out for each aggressive act vs. every two acts). A detailed discussion of specific types of fixed and variable rates of punishment is beyond the scope of this book. However, studies of different schedules of time-out administration have been set in educational or institutional environments under which painstaking behavioral data are recorded. Barring discussion of the complex details, it is important to note that inconsistent use of time-out can be somewhat effective. Further, gradual fading from a more consistent to less consistent schedule of time-out can maintain reduced rates of target behavior (Calhoun & Matherne, 1975; Greene et al., 1970). There are limits, however, as some research has found time-out to be ineffective when applied on a "thinner" schedule (e.g., given for every 4 instances of target behavior; Martin & Hasbrouck, 1977).

Take-away point: As with other forms of punishment, a consistent schedule in which each instance of a child's target behavior is followed immediately with time-out is most effective for reducing problem behavior. However, if consistency cannot be guaranteed or cannot be guaranteed in the long term, in many cases, time-out can still be effective in reducing and maintaining lower rates of problem behavior.

6.7 Release From Time-Out

Release contingencies related to time-out, or the criteria by which caregivers judge a child's time-out to be complete, can be thought of in three categories: time-based release, behavior-based release, or a combination of time- and behavior-based release.

6.7.1 Time-Based Release

This is a simple concept. A child spends a predetermined amount of time in time-out, and, regardless of behavior, the time-out ends on schedule. This means the child can scream, make inappropriate statements, kick, etc. while in time-out without penalty. Most nonexclusionary time-outs can operate under purely time-based release contingencies. To execute a nonexclusionary time-out, since caregivers need only to restrict access to reinforcers (e.g., toys, attention), there is less reason to require specific behavior from the child. For instance, the child could receive a time-out from sports play during gym class for 5 minutes.

Purely time-based release time-outs may be simpler for caregivers to administer than those that require a behavioral component. However, they have two disadvantages. First, some caregivers do not tolerate allowing a child to behave freely (e.g., scream, make a mess) during time-out, so a behavior-based release contingency may be warranted (e.g., sit quietly for 5 seconds). Second, time-outs with no behavioral release requirements may allow the child to avoid or escape an instruction. If a time-out is given for noncompliance, and there is no compliance requirement tied to release from time-out, time-out may actually be reinforcing (i.e., negative reinforcement associated with escape from the aversive task). In these cases, a child may prefer to have time-out over complying with instructions to do a nonpreferred task (e.g., start homework). Again, adding a behavior-based release contingency could increase the effectiveness of time-out in this situation.

Time-based time-outs may be simpler to administer

6.7.2 Behavior-Based Release

Behavior-based release gives children the advantage of feeling in control

In this configuration, time-out continues until a child performs or accomplishes a certain behavior. This contingency is at play when caregivers tell a child: "Go to your room. You can come out when you are calm," or "…when you are ready to apologize." Job card grounding, requiring completion of chore(s) before returning access to privileges, is also considered a behavior-based release procedure (see Chapter 3 for a description of job card grounding). With behavior-based release from time-out, the child experiences time-out from specified reinforcement only for the amount of time it takes for the child to complete the obligatory task. This format gives children the advantage of feeling in control of how long consequences last.

6.7.3 Time- and Behavior-Based Release

The combination of time- and behavior-based time-out release is often used in behavior therapy

Just as it sounds, this final release contingency combines time- and behavior-based requirements. Release contingencies for time-outs within many evidence-based behavior therapy programs operate this way. These programs often use a prescribed time-out duration (e.g., 3 minutes, 2 minutes for each year of the child's age) followed by a behavior-contingent release (e.g., 5–15 seconds of silence at the end of time-out; Barkley, 2013; Eyberg & Funderburk, 2011; McMahon & Forehand, 2003). This is called *contingent delay*. Behavioral contingencies for release following time-based criteria can be even more intricate. For instance, children who remain calm following a specific time-out duration may then be required to comply with a specific task once released from time-out in order to avoid returning to time-out. This might mean requiring reparations (e.g., apologizing) or following an instruction when noncompliance was the initial reason for time-out (e.g., put on your shoes).

In some time- and behavior-based release contingencies, time-out duration may be more precisely defined based on behavioral contingencies. In a study of the Children's Summer Treatment Program, Fabiano and colleagues (2004) employed an "escalating-deescalating time-out." Time-out started with a basic time-based release contingency (e.g., 5 minutes). Depending on the child's behavior, the time-out period could be made longer or shorter. Calmly accepting time-out for the first half led to a reduction of duration by half (i.e., 2.5 minutes), and aggressive behavior after being assigned to time-out resulted in adding 5 minutes to the time-out duration, up to 15-minutes. This improved time-out effectiveness for only 25% of children.

6.7.4 Comparing Release Contingencies

Both time-based and behavior-based time-outs are effective

Which type of release contingency is best? Some empirical evidence seems to show that, when it comes to overall effectiveness, it does not really matter. All available comparative studies on the topic found that both time-based and contingent delay time-outs were effective at reducing target behavior (Bean & Roberts, 1981; Day & Roberts, 1983; Donaldson & Vollmer, 2011; Erford, 1999; Fabiano et al., 2004; Hobbs & Forehand, 1975; Luiselli et al., 2006;

Mace et al., 1986). Only two studies showed relatively greater effectiveness for contingent delay time-outs over time-based time-outs (Erford, 1999; Hobbs & Forehand, 1975). One study showed greater efficacy for contingent delay release over purely behavior-based release (i.e., when children were "ready to comply"; Bean & Roberts, 1981). In support of time-based time-outs, Luiselli and colleagues (2006) found that time-based release contingencies resulted in less overall time in time-out, an important factor for many busy families and childcare staff. In support of behavior-based release, Hobbs and Forehand (1975) showed quicker improvements in target behavior under this condition than with purely time-based release.

Time-based release may result in shorter time-outs

While these studies provided evidence about how release contingencies influence the effectiveness of time-out on overall target behavior (e.g., noncompliance), what do we know about their impacts on disruptive behavior *during* time-out? Three studies have demonstrated that time-outs operating with behavioral release contingencies (i.e., staying calm for a portion of the time-out) significantly reduced, but did not eliminate, disruptive behavior *during* time-out when compared with purely time-based release contingencies (Donaldson & Vollmer, 2011; Erford, 1999; Hobbs & Forehand, 1975). In addition to decreased disruptive behavior during time-out as a goal in itself, Donaldson and Vollmer (2011) investigated the hypothesis that more disruptive behavior during time-out would be associated with greater disruptive behavior following time-out. This hypothesis was not supported.

Behavior-based time-outs may reduce disruptive behavior during time-out

Take-away point: Time-outs operating under a variety of release contingencies have consistently demonstrated effectiveness in reducing target behavior. Only a small proportion of the evidence has demonstrated superior effectiveness for improving target behavior by using contingent delay (e.g., requiring quiet behavior at the end of time-out) over purely time-based release contingencies. Similarly, only a small number of studies have shown comparatively less disruptive behavior *during* time-out itself for behavior contingent delay than time-based release time-outs. Therefore, because time-based release procedures are shorter lasting and less complicated to administer, they are likely to be appropriate in most cases.

6.8 Escape

Escape is a factor not explicitly delineated and discussed in much detail in several previous reviews of time-out parameters. Two forms of escape are relevant to this discussion: (1) escape from time-out itself, and (2) escape from other environmental stimuli as a function of time-out.

6.8.1 Escape *From* Time-Out

Many children are bound to escape the location or conditions of time-out if given the opportunity (Bean & Roberts, 1981). Theoretically, if time-out is effective at reducing target behavior by limiting access to reinforcement, and children regain access to reinforcement by escaping the conditions of time-out, it would follow that escape from time-out would limit its effectiveness. Research supports this (Roberts & Powers, 1990). As such, a variety of procedures to manage escape from time-out, sometimes referred to as back-up methods, have been developed. A recent review of the literature revealed that repeated put-backs, spanking, physical barriers (e.g., room time-out), and holding techniques were the most commonly reported back-up methods (Everett et al., 2007).

Back-up methods

The use of spanking continues to decline for a variety of reasons, and current research and behavioral parent training programs no longer recommend it as a back-up. Nevertheless, previous studies have shown equivalent effectiveness at improvement in target behavior (e.g., compliance) for barrier and spanking back-up methods (Day & Roberts, 1983; Roberts, 1988; Roberts & Powers, 1990). Barrier and spanking methods led to shorter time-outs than using no back-up for escape and showed relatively better effectiveness than a holding method (Roberts & Powers, 1990).

Spanking is not recommended as a back-up method

Research attention and clinical work has shifted away from spanking as a back-up. As an alternative, McNeil and colleagues (1994) tested the effectiveness of a two-chair hold procedure. The back-up procedure involved the caregiver sitting in a second chair behind the child's chair and using a 45-second modified basket hold. This procedure was effective, but, as with Roberts and Powers' (1990) results, it was less effective than spanking as a back-up. Additionally, holding the child required parental emotion regulation and was deemed inappropriate for parents with anger control problems who might inadvertently harm the child during restraint.

Two-chair hold procedure

Back-up methods that do not require touching the child are preferred as they minimize the potential for reinforcement through attention or sensory input (Magee & Ellis, 2001), physical aggression between caregiver and child, and certain ethical and legal violations in some settings (Nelson & Rutherford, 1983). Currently, barriers for escape (e.g., closing a gate, door to the child's room), extending time-out duration, restriction of privilege (i.e., response cost), and deferred time-outs are recommended as back-up procedures in programs such as The Defiant Children Program (Barkley, 2013), HNC (McMahon & Forehand, 2003), and PCIT (Eyberg & Funderburk, 2011). As used for escape, deferred time-outs involve removing caregiver attention and access to reinforcers until the child cooperates with time-out. Warzak and Floress (2009) demonstrated effectiveness with this method, and mothers have rated both deferred time-outs and barriers (e.g., room time-out) as acceptable back-up methods (Kunkle & Ortiz, 2016). If a suitable back-up method cannot be identified, behavior can be gradually shaped to accept time-out (Shriver & Allen, 1996). In this approach, children are put in time-out for very short periods and released before they attempt to escape, with time-out duration being increased over time to its desired length.

Back-up methods without touching the child are preferred

Gradual increase of time-out acceptance

6.8.2 Escape *Through* Time-Out

Caregivers and therapists should be wary of the possibility for time-out to function as a form of escape from nonpreferred environmental stimuli. As described in Chapter 2 regarding children with developmental disabilities, time-out may actually reinforce target behavior for some children who enjoy being removed from an overly stimulating environment. Likewise, time-out may serve as an escape from general social demands. For example, in time-out children can often freely engage in self-stimulatory behavior (Solnick et al., 1977). Across populations, time-out is highly likely to serve an escape function from caregiver demands. For instance, disruptive behavior of children in classroom settings who wish to discontinue difficult academic tasks is often inadvertently reinforced by sending the child out of the classroom to the principal's office or sensory room. In the same way, children can escape having to comply with a caregiver's instruction by refusing and "escaping" *to* time-out.

To avoid reinforcing noncompliance with escape, many behavioral parent training programs advocate instructional re-presentation following time-out for noncompliance. In other words, the child is required to comply with the original instruction to end the time-out procedure. Everett and colleagues (2007) investigated the relative efficacy of this method when noncompliance was maintained by escape. This important study challenged the idea that time-out should not be used to manage behavior maintained by escape, particularly in the case of children with autism spectrum disorder. Results showed that time-out with instructional re-presentation was much more effective than time-out without instructional re-presentation. However, even the latter was associated with some improvements in overall compliance. Still, other research has shown that time-out may not be appropriate for problem behavior maintained by escape. Taylor and Miller (1997) showed that time-out reinforced screaming and disruptive behavior in children with developmental disabilities when these behaviors were assessed to be maintained by escape during a teacher demand condition. On the other hand, in the same experiment, time-out *was* effective in reducing problem behavior for other children with disabilities when their behavior was maintained by attention.

Requiring compliance with original command may minimize reinforcement

Time-out may not be appropriate for problem behavior maintained by escape

Take-away point: Implementing procedures to stop children escaping *from* time-out are important to time-out's overall effectiveness. A variety of these back-up methods have demonstrated effectiveness, and those that can be carried out without touching the child are ideal. Available evidence suggests that some behavior maintained by escape (e.g., noncompliance) can be successfully targeted with time-out, especially when re-introducing the original instruction. However, time-out may actually reinforce other problem behavior maintained by escape (e.g., disruptive classroom behavior during challenging tasks) such that alternative strategies may need to be employed.

7

Controversial Issues Related to Time-Out

Parenting techniques in general are often controversial because they are simultaneously personal, emotionally salient, culturally based, and critical for child functioning. In addition, childrearing practices affect every person on the planet. As time-out in child behavior management has been studied and implemented widely for at least six decades, it is no surprise that time-out has become the source of some controversy. Many prominent parenting experts have raised concerns about time-out as a specific practice, within the class of punishment as a whole, and as part of a broad criticism of behavioral contingencies in parenting. In this chapter, we summarize some of the most frequently cited concerns with time-out in context. We also discuss ethical and legal considerations pertaining to time-out. The goal of this chapter is to elevate the scientific evidence related to the use of time-out above theory, so readers may be more objective about the pros and cons of its use.

7.1   Behavioral Parenting Approaches

Behavioral approaches alter the environment of the child before, during, and after target behavior

A vast literature related to behavioral parenting approaches supports effectiveness in improving child behavioral health outcomes. Simply defined, behavioral theory operates on the principle that human (and animal) behavior is best understood and managed through conditioning. In other words, what happens in an individual's environment before, during, and after a behavior impacts the likelihood that the behavior will occur again. While targeting many other factors, behavioral parenting approaches primarily focus on altering what happens in the environment immediately after a child engages in specific behavior. Among other strategies, caregivers are trained to systematically administer reinforcement (e.g., praise) and consequences (e.g., time-out) to shape behavior. Although research supports the use of behavioral principles as highly effective at managing and improving child behavior, several criticisms have been leveled against behavioral parenting approaches.

First, critics argue that behavioral approaches make caregiver love and acceptance contingent on behavior. However, there is no evidence to support that children feel less loved or accepted when rewards and consequences are tied to their behavior. There are data, however, pointing to the negative effects of certain types of consequences used in particularly damaging ways. For instance, yelling and harsh verbal punishments have been linked with

Yelling and harsh verbal punishment are linked with negative outcomes

childhood depression and conduct problems (Wang & Kenny, 2014). Corporal punishment is another example, described below. We do not condone these *forms* of punishment. However, evidence does support the use of other forms of punishment, when necessary, within an overall model of frequent positive reinforcement. In fact, behavioral approaches to parenting are linked with decreases in the likelihood of caregivers engaging in other harmful strategies (e.g., physical abuse; Chaffin et al., 2011) and decreases in the likelihood of negative outcomes (e.g., substance use, antisocial behavior, mental health problems; Kaminski & Claussen, 2017).

> Behavioral approaches may decrease harmful strategies and increase positive outcomes

Behavioral approaches clearly support the idea of directing reinforcement and consequences toward a child's behavior rather than the child. Caregivers are encouraged to label behavior as specifically as possible to communicate this concept to children (e.g., "I am proud of the way you followed directions"; "Because you made a mess, the paint will be put away for the rest of the day"). Moreover, it would be difficult to parent without using reinforcement and consequences. This would mean never offering specific praise for children's achievements and never administering natural consequences for dangerous behavior (e.g., removing a knife from a toddler who is waving it around). After all, much of our society's behavior is regulated by behavioral principles. Working at a job earns many people a salary, and breaking some laws results in financial penalties. Children may naturally gain friends by engaging in prosocial behavior and lose them by being aggressive. Using behavioral strategies for child behavior management is simply an extension of natural and societal patterns, which may help prepare children to function in the outside world. Lastly, not all reinforcement must be assigned to target behaviors when using behavioral parenting approaches. Affection, gifts, and positive interactions can and should be offered freely, independently of behavior. Behavioral principles are simply available for strategic use when caregivers wish to increase or decrease specific behavior.

Second, concerns that behavioral approaches undermine individuals' *intrinsic motivation* have been raised. This idea became widespread in the 1980s. Social psychology theorists proposed that a force called *intrinsic interest* dictates the likelihood that an individual engages in a behavior, independent of environmental input (Deci & Ryan, 1985). The intrinsic motivation literature comprises many studies showing that when individuals are rewarded externally (e.g., paid, socially recognized) for engaging in behavior, and at some point in the future rewards are discontinued, individuals engage in that behavior less than when it was being rewarded. Behavioral psychologists have found fault with these studies and the overall theory of intrinsic motivation. Flora (1990) argued that intrinsic motivation research: (1) rarely measures baseline levels of behavior, (2) discounts environmental antecedents of intrinsically interesting behavior (e.g., a teacher calling an activity a "test" vs. a "puzzle"), (3) mistakenly assumes that all rewards are always reinforcing, and (4) relies too much on theory and constructs that cannot directly be measured. In addition to flawed research, counter-examples exist to negate the idea that externally reinforcing behavior hurts internal motivation. For instance, cigarette smoking is initially extrinsically (i.e., socially) motivated but becomes intrinsically motivated over time (Flora, 1990).

> Intrinsic motivation and interest

> Flaws within intrinsic motivation research

Children's intrinsic motivation to behave prosocially

The risk of damaging a child's internal motivation to engage in prosocial behavior by using rewards is prevalent in mainstream parenting as well. In our clinical experiences, caregivers frequently raise concerns that praising their children for doing things they should be expected to do (e.g., keeping their rooms clean) will make them dependent on praise rather than being motivated by the satisfaction of completing the task itself. In his popular book, *Punished by Rewards: The Trouble with Gold Stars, Incentive Plans, A's, Praise, and Other Bribes* (1993), Alfie Kohn characterized behavioral parenting as manipulating children into behaving in certain ways in the short term and argued that this has long-term negative effects on intrinsic motivation. Kohn proposed that relying on reinforcement and punishment to motivate behavior decreases creativity and risk-taking behavior. Especially related to educational settings, Kohn advocated for more collaboration, choice, and modified course content to increase intrinsic interest in learning.

While these arguments may sound convincing and the alternatives appealing, there must be sound evidence to back them up. In response to Kohn (1993), Reitman's (1998) critical review, "Punished by Misunderstanding," pointed out that even research supporting collaborative learning approaches shows that academic success is achieved in concert with external individual and group rewards. The alternative approaches championed by Kohn did not have convincing evidence indicating greater effects on academic achievement (Reitman, 1998). Finally, little evidence either for or against long-term negative consequences of externally rewarding behavior on internal motivation exists (Reitman, 1998).

Little evidence related to negative consequences of rewards

Despite the various definitions, variables, and constructs under investigation in these domains, caregivers and experts have the same goals for children: both short- and long-term healthy development and functioning. Ideally, children would consistently initiate and maintain desirable behavior without any formalized intervention from the outside world. However, when they do not, overwhelming empirical evidence suggests that behavioral methods help. Although it is easy to imagine that using behavioral methods to motivate children's behavior could be damaging or transient, research does not support these assumptions. Later in this chapter we highlight ethical and legal considerations related to withholding evidence-based treatment without evidence-based rationale.

7.2 Punishment

Similar to concerns that behavioral strategies overall may have negative effects, the concept of punishment has been questioned and criticized in many circles of modern parenting. When browsing bookstores, magazines, and the internet for information on parenting, one quickly encounters titles such as, *Parenting Without Punishment*, *Gentle Parenting*, and *No Spanking, No Time-Out, No Problems*. While it is well-known that authoritarian parenting, characterized by high control and low warmth (Baumrind, 1967), is associated with negative child outcomes, this message has more recently evolved to the increasingly popular notion that all punishment is harmful to children.

Growing concern that all types of punishment are harmful to children

7.2.1 What Is Punishment?

Despite the fact that many claims about punishment have developed from a variety of other fields and theoretical orientations, it is important to understand its original scientific definition, which comes from the behavioral literature. B. F. Skinner (1953) defined *punishment* as a procedure involving either removal of reinforcement or introduction of an aversive stimulus, resulting in a decrease in a contingent behavior. For instance, removing the possibility of eating dessert (i.e., reinforcement) and lecturing about poor nutrition (i.e., aversive stimulus) after a child refuses to eat their vegetables are considered forms of punishment, *if and only if* they are followed by decreased vegetable refusal in the future. If withholding dessert and lecturing resulted in increased refusal to eat vegetables in the future, these consequences would fall into the category of reinforcement, not punishment, regardless of whether they appeared to be punishing. Behaviorally speaking, punishment does not refer to a group of negative consequences intended to inflict suffering. This misconception likely contributes to the popular belief that all punishment is bad. In its scientific definition, punishment is defined only by the subsequent decrease in the likelihood of a target behavior in the future. For example, if a child blows a whistle repeatedly indoors, both ignoring the noise and taking the whistle away from the child for one minute would be considered punishments *if* they reduced indoor whistle blowing in the future; however, it would be difficult to argue that either scenario constitutes suffering. Likewise, it is difficult to imagine an approach to parenting that could operate without the use of any form of punishment, as parents must frequently discourage certain types of behavior (e.g., unsafe behavior).

Definition by B. F. Skinner

Punishment is not intended to inflict suffering

Scientific definition of punishment

7.2.2 Concerns With Punishment

Punishment is often misunderstood and thought of negatively, but what are the specific arguments against it? Some have argued against the use of punishment altogether, characterizing it as overly cruel and harsh. Others believe the side effects or negative consequences of implementing punishment procedures are too great. Still others have contended that punishment is ineffective, only providing a temporary solution to behavior problems. We outline each of these arguments as well as related evidence and theory.

Cruelty

Throughout the history of behaviorism, punishment has been alternately labeled as cruel and defended as useful and humane (Solomon, 1964). *Cruelty* is defined by Merriam-Webster as the intentional infliction of pain or suffering devoid of humane feelings, while *humane* is defined as marked by compassion, sympathy, or consideration for humans or animals. These definitions help clarify the issue somewhat, but classification of cruelty is still subjective. It is clear that a variety of punishing stimuli (e.g., corporal punishment, criticism) *could* be used in ways that meet the definition of cruel and inhumane. For example, the use of physical discipline or corporal punishment has been a popular method of punishing children (and adults) throughout history. By

Definition

definition, corporal punishment is intended to inflict pain. The involvement of consideration for human feelings or compassion is another matter. Regarding child behavior management, the goal of punishment is to discourage or decrease future negative behavior (e.g., aggression, elopement). This alone may be interpreted as consideration and compassion for the child. However, not all punishment is delivered in ways that demonstrate such care and compassion. Therefore, punishment in all its forms should neither be blindly accepted as justified nor rejected as cruel.

National and international organizations have recently begun condemning corporal punishment (American Academy of Pediatrics; AAP, 1998; 2018; Global Initiative to End All Corporal Punishment of Children, 2020a; 2020b). A crucial distinction should be made here about the basis of these recommendations. The condemnation of corporal punishment by these organizations is not based on popular opinion or specific theories. Instead, the position statements were disseminated because there is substantial *evidence* to support these claims. Meta-analyses and longitudinal research studies from around the world have demonstrated that corporal punishment is associated with negative mental health outcomes, poorer caregiver–child relationships, increased aggression, antisocial behavior, and physical abuse (AAP, 2018; Gershoff, 2002; Gershoff & Bitensky, 2007). At the same time, even this body of research does not suggest that every incidence of spanking, for example, is cruel and will harm children in all circumstances. However, there is substantial evidence that the risks associated with spanking clearly outweigh benefits. This research also highlights the detrimental effects of the specific technique (i.e., aggressive infliction of physical pain) rather than the function of punishment as a whole (i.e., decreasing undesirable behavior).

Specific punishment procedures, as currently advocated by behavioral parent training approaches, including time-out, are designed with great compassion and consideration for human feelings while aimed at minimizing distress. In addition to the potential risks related to punishment, we must consider the potential positive effects. The inherent challenge in the ethical treatment of others is to produce the most good while doing the least harm. Given the overwhelming evidence base related to the positive outcomes of behavioral methods, it would be a disservice to abandon these treatments based on theoretical arguments. However, it is important that research and clinical practice continue to examine the evidence related to its methods to provide maximum benefits with minimal risk.

Side Effects of Punishment

Along with the potential for cruelty in administration, theorists and researchers have argued the potential for negative side effects of punishment. Proposed undesirable side effects have included increased aggression, extinction bursts, escape or avoidance, and countercontrol.

Aggression

As noted in our review of the corporal punishment literature, certain punishment techniques have been associated with increased aggression (Gershoff, 2002). In addition to the possibility of modeling aggression through physical discipline (Bandura et al., 1961), there is evidence of "punishment-induced aggression" related to nonaggressive punishment (Sidman, 1989). Animal studies have shown that, when presented with aversive stimuli (e.g., shock), animals sometimes become aggressive toward other animals and objects (Ulrich & Azrin, 1962; Ulrich et al., 1964). Longer lasting, higher intensity, more frequent aversive stimuli were associated with more aggression in animals (Ulrich & Azrin, 1962; Ulrich et al., 1964). Further, individual variables (e.g., species, sex) and environmental factors (e.g., space, hunger) influenced the likelihood of aggression. In their review of human subjects research, Fontes and Shahan (2020) noted that punishment-induced aggression has only been observed in response to physical punishment. In addition, authors explain that aversive stimuli in the animal research was response-independent, and therefore could not even be considered a form of punishment. In conclusion, upon further examination of the evidence, concern for punishment-induced aggression in humans using nonphysical forms of punishment like time-out is low.

Punishment-induced aggression in response to physical punishment

Nonphysical forms of punishment have not been linked to aggression

Extinction Bursts

Extinction bursts provide another possible mechanism for aggression related to punishment. Extinction occurs when reinforcement for a behavior is discontinued (Katz & Lattal, 2021). For instance, a teacher uses extinction when she discontinues calling on a child who shouts out an answer rather than raising their hand. An extinction burst is defined as a temporary increase in responding at the onset of extinction (Katz & Lattal, 2021). In our example, the child might temporarily increase the frequency or intensity with which they holler out as soon as the teacher discontinues responding. Many variables determine whether and to what extent extinction bursts occur in different situations (Katz & Lattal, 2021). For example, an extinction burst may involve aggression. This can occur if aggression in particular is the target behavior that is no longer being reinforced. However, extinction bursts may implicate a variety of undesirable behavior that caregivers no longer wish to reinforce (e.g., whining, throwing objects, name calling). In our clinical experience, extinction bursts are quite common when caregivers first begin ignoring a child's minor misbehavior. Nevertheless, caregivers can be warned to anticipate this and prepared to manage it. We find that caregivers handle this transition much more calmly and confidently when they know it will be short-lived. When compared with continuing to reinforce an unwanted behavior over time, an anticipated, short-term extinction burst is usually preferable.

Definition

Escape and Avoidance

Escape and avoidance are both relevant to punishment. Escape occurs when exposure to an aversive stimulus is discontinued, while avoidance occurs when exposure to an aversive stimulus is prevented. To illustrate, a child who covers their ears while being yelled at for spilling milk is escaping the yelling. A child who covers the milk with his plate to prevent being yelled at for spilling is avoiding the yelling.

It is easy to imagine that punishment delivered in the form of aversive stimuli would be likely to induce escape or avoidance. A common example involves children experiencing soiling accidents. If children are punished for soiling (e.g., scolded by a parent), they are more likely to hide the accident next time (i.e., avoid) or deny having an accident when confronted (i.e., escape). For these reasons, scolding for soiling accidents is not recommended. When using punishment for child behavior management, the potential for escape and avoidance should be taken into account. In our experience, children often attempt to avoid or escape punishment when sent to time-out. In many situations, child avoidance of time-out can be used to the family's advantage. For example, children can be taught to engage in specific positive behavior to avoid punishment (e.g., follow directions after a warning statement is given) or escape punishment (e.g., sitting quietly to be released from the chair). While escape and avoidance are inevitable to some degree, evidence supporting the use of punishment within larger behavioral approaches suggests that their effects can be successfully mitigated (Kaminski et al., 2008).

> **Allowing avoidance of punishment may reinforce positive behavior**

To be clear, although escape and avoidance are possible reactions to punishment, discounting all punishment strategies simply to prevent escape and avoidance would be misguided. The conscientious use of punishment techniques as part of a larger, positive behavioral approach means that other strategies are employed first. As such, caregivers should learn to provide positive reinforcement for alternative behavior (e.g., giving a treat for toileting appropriately) whenever possible rather than relying on punishment as the primary response.

Countercontrol

> **Definition**

Another concern related to punishment is the idea of countercontrol. Countercontrol can be thought of as an individual's attempt to extinguish or punish a punisher's behavior in a socially aversive situation (Sidman, 1989; Skinner, 1953). In several studies, human beings have demonstrated behavior attributed to countercontrol (e.g., aggression, resistance, or escape) in response to high levels of punishment aimed at social control (Sidman, 1989; Skinner, 1953). Although the validity of research evidence in this domain has been called into question (Fontes & Shahan, 2020), theoretical connections can be drawn between countercontrol, the coercive family process (Patterson, 1979), and symptoms of children with oppositional defiant disorder. In each, undesirable child behavior is likely to be perpetuated by overly punitive dynamics.

> **Minimizing punishment lowers the risk of invoking countercontrol**

To minimize the risk of invoking countercontrol, the coercive cycle, and oppositional defiant behavior in general, caregivers and therapists should minimize unnecessary punishment. This may mean relying on a variety of other complementary strategies and using punishment only when other measures (e.g., positive reinforcement) are insufficient. As highlighted throughout this book, punishment is one tool within a larger context of positive reinforcement and positive caregiver–child interactions. It is certainly likely that if used too frequently, with great intensity, and/or for long durations, punishment will incite negative effects related to countercontrol, oppositional defiance, and the coercive process. In our clinical experience, this occurs in many families who seek treatment for a variety of oppositional and defiant behavior problems. While the goal with these families is to increase the ratio of positive to negative interactions, this does not mean that all punishment must be discontinued. When used thoughtfully, punishment strategies such as planned ignoring and time-out can be appropriate for nearly every family.

Indeed, even proponents of BPT caution against relying heavily on punishment. In all major BPT programs, punishment is introduced as secondary to positive reinforcement techniques (Reitman & McMahon, 2013). For example, ignoring a child's minor misbehavior for a few seconds is considered a mild form of punishment as the reinforcer of a caregiver's attention is removed. However, this technique is only effective in the context of high levels of caregiver reinforcement in the caregiver–child relationship. In BPT programs, punishment strategies are introduced gradually, are to be used sparingly, and are only recommended in the context of positive parenting skills. Meta-analytic data suggests that punishment is necessary but not sufficient for behavior management (Kaminski et al., 2008).

In BPT punishment is secondary to positive reinforcement techniques

Punishment is necessary but not sufficient for behavior management

Temporary Effects

Finally, it has been argued that punishment decreases the likelihood of target behavior in the short-term, but the effect is only temporary. Sidman (1989) cited several animal studies and one human study demonstrating that when punished, target behavior only temporarily decreased before returning to baseline levels. In a counter argument, Fontes and Shahan (2020) cited several other studies in which reduced responding due to punishment persisted. For instance, McMillan (1967) showed that time-out produced longer lasting target behavior suppression than did electric shock, using squirrel monkeys. Depending on various factors, therefore, the duration of punishment effects varies.

Decreased effectiveness

Controlled studies regarding this issue differ from real-world settings in an important way. In real-world settings, punishment is inextricable from other sources of reinforcement in the environment. While ignoring may only temporarily decrease aggression for a child attempting to access candy in a laboratory environment, in a real-world setting, caregivers may simultaneously teach an alternative response (e.g., asking nicely) which can be reinforced. It is unlikely, then, that when caregivers consistently punish aggression and consistently reinforce asking nicely, a child would quickly return to aggression when punishment ceases. With this in mind, the potentially temporary effects of punishment should not be thought of in a vacuum when considering their use in applied settings.

In real-world settings, caregivers can reinforce alternative responses while discouraging negative responses

7.3 Controversies Around Time-Out

As with behavioral approaches and punishment as a whole, critics have argued that time-out is an artificial form of motivation and that it can be experienced as overly harsh or damaging. A summary of the most frequently cited concerns specific to time-out and their counterarguments are presented, namely that time-out traumatizes children, damages them psychologically and physiologically, or has otherwise negative long-term effects. We then examine a commonly proposed alternative to time-out and punishment called *exclusively positive parenting*. Finally, research around time-out acceptability is reviewed.

7.3.1 Does Time-Out Cause Trauma and Physiological Harm?

Concerns with emotional suffering

While time-out is not physically painful, and often is recommended as an alternative to physical discipline (AAP, 2018), concerns have been raised about the potential for children to experience emotional suffering while in time-out. Some have claimed that time-out itself is traumatizing or highly likely to re-traumatize a child who has been abused or neglected in the past. Proponents of these arguments frequently cite a study published in *Science*, which showed that brain activity during social exclusion resembles brain activity experienced during physical pain (Eisenberger et al., 2003). Brain scans showed that similar brain regions and activation patterns occurred during physical pain, implicit exclusion, and explicit exclusion. Implicit exclusion occurred when participants were not allowed to join a virtual ball tossing game because of "technical difficulties," and explicit exclusion occurred when they could not join because other virtual players did not toss the ball to them. Only during explicit, and not implicit exclusion, did another region of the brain become active to help participants regulate their emotions and behavior. In their conclusions, authors interpreted this positively, as the brain is "alerting us when we have sustained injury to our social connections, allowing restorative measures to be taken" (Eisenberger et al., 2003, p. 292).

No indication that time-out outcomes are similar to outcomes of physical discipline

It makes sense that the brain would respond along similar pathways to discomfort, either physical or social. As Eisenberger and colleagues pointed out, the function of both processes is likely related to helping human beings learn and behave differently in the future to avoid such distress. Nowhere in this research is it stated or implied that all social discomfort or exclusion is severely painful, only that the same brain regions and activation patterns are implicated (Eisenberger et al., 2003). Likewise, the results do *not* indicate that the outcomes of time-out are in any way similar to the negative outcomes of physical discipline. Furthermore, this study provides no evidence about any connection between social exclusion by peers and exclusion from positive reinforcement by caregivers in the context of time-out.

No evidence of a connection between social exclusion and exclusion from reinforcement

Results of this same study were mischaracterized in 2014 when *Time* published an article entitled, "Time-Outs are Hurting Your Child" (Siegel & Bryson, 2014). The *Time* article argued that time-out constitutes isolation and rejection. Authors were concerned that time-out sends children the message that when they are distressed, they should be made to "suffer alone" and that brain activity experienced during emotional pain is similar to that of physical abuse (Siegel & Bryson, 2014). The article received much national attention from other media outlets, caregivers, and psychologists alike.

Importantly, Siegel and Bryson later released a clarification (Siegel, 2014). In it, they noted that *Time* had used the title, "Time-Outs are Hurting Your Children" without permission, which had led to confusion. They also noted that research demonstrated connections between time-out and physical *pain* not child abuse, which the magazine had reportedly misrepresented. Siegel and Bryson went on to clarify that it is only the inappropriate use of what they term a "punitive time-out" (i.e., frequent, prolonged, and coupled with parent anger) which they do not condone. Siegel and Bryson themselves stated that they are "all for" the use of appropriate time-outs (i.e., delivered calmly and infrequently) and cited the "extensive" research supporting this practice (Siegel, 2014).

These two articles highlight important issues related to parenting and the media as a whole. Too often, catchy headlines and fearmongering target caregivers to generate buzz, attention, clicks, and sales. In this pursuit, the true scientific evidence is lost. In fact, Drayton and colleagues (2014) found that none of the 100 most searched websites discussing time-out contained complete and accurate information. It is important that professionals responsibly consume scientific literature and pass findings along to families. Now, more than ever, families are vulnerable to faulty guidance about child behavior management.

Majority of websites contain incomplete and inaccurate information on time-out

In response to misleading popular media publications on time-out, psychological researchers have published articles defending the evidence base behind time-out (Dadds & Tully, 2019; Quetsch et al. 2015, 2017). These articles responded to claims that time-out procedures can traumatize or re-traumatize children with histories of abuse or neglect. Quetsch and colleagues (2017) contrasted the definitions of traumatizing and re-traumatizing events with children's experiences in time-out. Key components of trauma include exposure to real or imagined physical or psychological danger. These authors argued that being told to sit in a chair for a minimum of 3 minutes does not likely constitute a trauma experience. Accordingly, there is no scientific evidence demonstrating behavioral or emotional symptoms of trauma related to time-out. This applies to time-outs involving a back-up room as well.

Responses to concerns about time-out traumatizing children

No scientific evidence relates symptoms of trauma to time-out

While it is easy to imagine that children with abuse or neglect histories would somehow be damaged by feeling upset during behavioral limit-setting, this is an unsupported concern. In fact, by imposing behavioral limits, specifically when using time-out, evidence indicates that families are less likely to resort to harmful methods of discipline (e.g., yelling, punishing with anger, using physical discipline; Chaffin et al., 2011; Kaminski & Claussen, 2017). In turn, children who can rely on caregivers' use of calm, consistent, predictable time-out procedures have demonstrated improvements in symptoms of anxiety, emotion dysregulation, and trauma (Chronis-Tuscano et al., 2015; Lieneman et al., 2020; Pearl et al., 2012). For those who still have concerns, adaptations to the use of a back-up room have been made for children with maltreatment histories involving isolation or confinement. These adaptations include restricting a privilege instead or having a caregiver accompany the child to the back-up room (Quetsch et al., 2017).

Caregivers less likely to use harmful discipline methods

Adaptations for children with isolation or confinement histories

7.3.2 Are There Other Negative Outcomes Associated With Time-Out?

As discussed in relation to punishment as a class, theoretical concerns that time-out causes undesirable side effects are prevalent (Gartrell 2001; 2002; Schreiber, 1999). Some concerned caregivers and professionals worry that children will not learn to express their emotions properly if time-out is used for aggressive or disruptive behavior. Others argue that children will not learn how to problem solve or behave appropriately if they are simply put in time-out. Finally, some have contended that time-out creates a negative, problem-focused environment which could increase overall levels of children's aggression.

Time-Out as Part of a Larger Intervention

Time-out is not recommended as a standalone intervention

The most important point to consider when evaluating these arguments is that time-out is not recommended as a standalone parenting or educational intervention. It should always be used as a part of a larger, positive reinforcement-based approach in the context of positive caregiver–child interactions. Moreover, caregivers do not have to choose between promoting desirable behavior (e.g., guidance, problem solving, supportive relationships) and discouraging undesirable behavior (e.g., discipline, time-out).

Many of the theoretically based arguments against time-out are built on poor understanding of behavioral principles. For example, some mistakenly assume that time-out is meant for children to think about their actions (Schreiber, 1999; Ucci, 1998). On the contrary, reflection during time-out is unnecessary. In fact, time-out originated from effective use with a variety of nonhuman species with little capacity for "thoughts" (e.g., rats, pigeons). In another misinterpretation of behavioral principles, Ucci (1998) advocated for time-out but that caregivers not think of it as punishment. More accurately, any action, by definition, is a punishment if it causes a decrease in the behavior it follows. Lastly, many classroom management approaches, sometimes termed *guidance approaches,* advocate supportive, problem-solving conversations with children to decrease "mistaken behavior" over punishments like time-out (Gartrell, 1994). While these conversations likely promote positive development, there are two problems with this recommendation: (1) Positive problem-solving strategies and time-out are not mutually exclusive, and (2) if guidance approaches are effective in decreasing "mistaken behavior," they are, by definition, punishments. A risk of guidance approaches is that reasoning during negative attention seeking behaviors could inadvertently reinforce the misbehavior by providing immediate caregiver attention.

Expressing Emotions

For professionals and caregivers who want to help children express their emotions properly, these skills should be taught using modeling, practice, and reinforcement regardless of whether time-out is added or not. In fact, several BPT interventions explicitly focus on labeling emotions, coaching emotion regulation, and expressing empathy for children's distress (Chronis-Tuscano et al., 2016; Girard et al., 2018; Lenze et al., 2011). Time-out simply serves as an adjunct to discourage inappropriate communication strategies (e.g., hitting to request attention) and expressions of emotion (e.g., swearing when frustrated). This does not preclude using other skill-building or emotion processing techniques.

Problem Solving

Adults should engage in problem-solving conversations

As with expressing emotions, parents and teachers should engage in problem-solving conversations independent of times when children behave inappropriately. Given a supportive caregiver–child relationship in which appropriate behavior is already being reinforced, time-out simply discourages poor choices. Imagine a metaphorical fork in a child's path. When upset or frustrated, a child may have several paths to resolution, for example, asking for help, walking away, or hitting another child. While the child may have been taught the other adaptive, problem-solving strategies, hitting can be an easy, instinctive option. Using time-out does not preclude other teaching and problem-solving strategies, it simply blocks the path to inappropriate choices, making them less likely. In turn, children are then more motivated to choose an adaptive path, practicing positive skills they have learned and increasing odds of "getting it right" in the future. This concept is born out in the literature, as BPTs using time-out have greater positive impacts on children's behavior than those without it (Kaminski et al., 2008).

Time-out does not preclude other teaching and problem-solving strategies

Aggression and Negativity

In addition to concerns that time-out will undermine efforts to increase positive behavior, some fear that time-out will increase problems with aggression or increase negativity between caregivers and children. According to the literature, the direct opposite is true. Evidence supporting the use of interventions involving time-out to decrease aggression is overwhelming (Eyberg et al., 2008). In contrast with use of physical discipline, yelling, and even expressing disappointment, time-out was not associated with increases in children's aggression in a sample spanning six countries (Gershoff et al., 2010). As noted previously, evidence of punishment-induced aggression in humans is linked with physical punishment only (Fontes & Shahan, 2020). In line with extinction bursts, however, target behavior (e.g., aggression) has been shown to increase with initial time-outs but decrease with consistent use (see Brantner & Doherty, 1983; Fontes & Shahan, 2020 for reviews of the literature). In fact, Forcino and colleagues (2019) showed that time-out back-up procedures could feasibly and effectively decrease oppositional responding to time-out in older children.

Interventions with time-out may decrease aggression

Concerns that time-out will increase focus on negative child behavior or incite negativity in the caregiver–child relationship are neither supported by behavioral theory nor evidence. Behavioral theory holds that time-out functions by decreasing attention for negative behavior and creating contrast by reinforcing positive behavior. By definition, families who implement time-out properly are creating a less negative, more positive environment. Scientific evidence supports this theory. Behavioral parenting interventions using time-out have demonstrated strong evidence of reducing caregiver–child interaction problems, decreasing parenting stress, and increasing positive parenting practices (Eyberg et al., 2008).

No evidence that time-out increases focus on negative child behavior

7.3.3 Time-Out is Efficacious in Research, but Is It Effective in the "Real World"?

Though research supports time-out as a tightly controlled behavioral intervention, professionals often assume that time-out cannot be carried out with fidelity and consistency by caregivers in the "real world." Following this logic, real-world time-outs are expected to be ineffective at managing child behavior. Indeed, many families use time-out inappropriately or ineffectively on their own. Clinically, during pre-treatment assessments, we see many caregivers inadvertently reinforce negative behavior before, during, and after time-out by providing one-on-one attention (e.g., discussing the child's misbehavior at length). Other families use time-out too frequently, angrily, or unpredictably.

Common mistakes in time-out implementation

Environmental limitations and other demands on caregivers make it difficult to carry out time-out perfectly and consistently at all times. A traditional chair time-out may not be feasible when a parent is rushing out the door to get to work on time. Likewise, it can be quite difficult to manage a child's escape from time-out while a mother is nursing the child's sibling or while a teacher is supervising 20 other students. Accordingly, some of the BPT literature indicates that treatment success is moderated by socioeconomic factors (Lundahl et al., 2006) while some refutes this (Weeland et al., 2018).

Caregivers can learn to carry out strategies effectively and with fidelity

Despite these limitations, there is no evidence to suggest that parents or other nonprofessional caregivers cannot learn to administer time-out effectively or that effectiveness requires perfect fidelity. First, some caregivers use time-out effectively with no guidance at all. Their administration may be flawed by behavioral research standards, but overall, children learn to respect their caregiver's limits, nonetheless. For cases in which time-out does not reduce target behavior, professionals (e.g., psychologists, behavior analysts) can help. BPT programs that incorporate time-out typically instruct and sometimes coach caregivers to administer time-out in clinic, initially. The majority of practice, however, takes place independently at home. Weekly check-ins during session, observations, and/or videos are used to help caregivers refine home-based time-out procedures and ensure a concurrently high ratio of positive reinforcement. Ongoing at-home practice is fundamental to the strong literature base supporting BPT approaches (Kaminski & Claussen, 2017). Much of this literature reflects community-based effectiveness outcomes measured long after families have left treatment, indicating that whatever level of fidelity caregivers use is "good enough" in many cases (Hood & Eyberg, 2003).

Time-out is highly effective when administered by nonprofessionals in nonclinical settings

Research shows that time-out is highly effective even when administered by nonprofessionals in nonclinical settings. Wahler (1969) established that child behavior improvements demonstrated in clinic generalized to the home environment when caregivers implemented time-out at home. Forcino and colleagues (2019) concluded that, even with older children who strongly opposed imposition of consequences by adults, observational and caregiver reports indicated at-home feasibility and effectiveness of time-out. While expert administration of rigorous time-out protocols can be beneficial, overall, caregiver-administered time-out in the "real world," especially with training, can be highly effective as well.

7.3.4 Does Time-Out Only Affect Immediate Behavior Problems?

Some popular parenting authors have asserted that time-out only results in immediate compliance or behavior change without concern for long-term outcomes in the caregiver–child relationship or child development (Parent Effectiveness Training; Gordon, 2000; Kohn, 1993; Solter, 1998). This assumption implies that time-out and its immediate impact on behavior do not help and may even harm relationships and development. These authors correctly point out that the primary goal of time-out is to improve short-term compliance and behavior problems. They incorrectly assume that behavior management with time-out neither targets nor benefits other long-term outcomes.

In reality, time-out is linked with more than short-term behavior improvements. First, long-term behavioral improvements have been measured following time-out implementation (Baum & Forehand, 1981; Hood & Eyberg, 2003; Lavigueur et al., 1973; Long et al., 1994). In addition, children who abide by caregivers' behavioral limits (i.e., the short-term goal of time-out) experience a variety of developmental benefits. These caregivers have greater cooperation from their children in developing healthy habits around toilet training, sleep, nutrition, communication, academics, and social relationships. These children are less likely to have problems in the future related to substance abuse, mental health problems, and criminal activity (APA, 2013). The cascading effects of success in behavioral limit setting are nearly limitless.

> **Time-out is linked to long-term behavior improvements**
>
> **Behavioral limits facilitate development of other healthy habits**

In addition, evidence on time-out and BPT programs that incorporate it strongly supports improvements in caregiver–child relationships, parenting stress, and emotion regulation (Eyberg et al., 2008; Lieneman et al., 2020). Furthermore, parenting without effective discipline strategies (e.g., time-out) can lead to poor outcomes through permissive parenting (Baumrind, 1967). Time-out provides a vehicle for many families to achieve the ideal authoritative parenting style (Baumrind, 1967), a balance between high levels of warmth and control. Finally, no negative long-term outcomes of time-out have been identified (Knight et al., 2020).

> **No negative long-term outcomes of time-out have been identified**

7.3.5 Is Exclusively Positive Parenting Preferable to Time-Out?

A few "positive" parenting systems, like Parenting Effectiveness Training (PET) and Aware Parenting, advocate using no punishment whatsoever, expressly discouraging time-out and other "artificial" consequences (Gordon, 2000; Solter, 1998). Such exclusively positive parenting (EPP) programs and attachment parenting models follow the principle that if a caregiver responds sensitively, meets the emotional needs of the child, or engages in preventive problem solving, problem behaviors will simply decrease on their own. Proponents of the EPP movement argue that time-out is a punitive procedure that may control behavior problems in the short term but does not teach children how to manage conflict effectively or communicate about their feelings. These programs often advocate for a time-out alternative in which caregivers physically comfort, encourage discussion of feelings, and listen supportively. This concept is commonly referred to as time-in and is used as a direct alternative to time-out. This should not be confused with time-in described by many popular BPT programs which involves making everyday interactions more reinforcing. Although various experts behind EPP approaches have advanced degrees in psychology or medicine, typically, their claims are based largely on theory rather than substantial empirical evidence.

> **Claims typically based on theory rather than evidence**

At the time of this writing, six empirical studies had been published indicating causal effectiveness of EPP approaches for child behavior management (for a review, see Larzelere et al., 2020). These studies were based on four datasets investigating either an emotion coaching program (Tuning into Kids,

> **Studies on EPP programs**

TIK; Havighurst et al., 2013) or Collaborative and Proactive Solutions (CPS; Greene, 1998). TIK helps families of preschool age children and older learn to recognize, validate, and negotiate limits related to emotions. TIK has demonstrated large effects for improvements in emotion coaching and child behavior problems using a sample of children with externalizing behavior problems (Havighurst et al., 2013). CPS targets problem behavior in older children through three separate approaches (plans A, B, and C). Time-out would be considered part of plan A, the imposition of adult will and consequences. The goal of CPS is to decrease reliance on plan A and build skills in plan B, collaborative problem solving. Plan B should not be used in the heat of the moment when problem behavior occurs, but in advance, to prevent it (Greene, 1998). Ollendick and colleagues (2016) showed that, in a sample of 7 to 14-year-olds with oppositional defiant disorder, CPS produced comparable results to Barkley's parent management training approach (which includes time-out). Notably, CPS requires that children have the developmental abilities to engage in collaborative problems solving.

Similarities between EPP and BPT programs

While EPP programs and BPT programs using time-out have been pitted against one another, they need not be. Both are focused on helping children make more appropriate choices, increasing positive behavior, and preventing future behavior problems. EPP programs target these goals by engaging in preventive problem solving and targeting lagging skills (e.g., emotion recognition). BPT programs also target lagging skills (e.g., compliance, self-regulation) by engaging families in graduated practice. Further, BPT programs prevent future behavior problems by increasing motivation to engage in adaptive responses, thereby increasing practice and skill related to appropriate behavior. Both approaches encourage using high ratios of positive (e.g., praise, empathy) to negative (e.g., commands) skills.

Differences between EPP and BPT programs

It seems, however, that the modus operandi of each approach has been oversimplified by proponents of the other. Behaviorists often view EPP programs as advocating for no behavioral limits at all. More accurately, even CPS and TIK concede that behavioral limits, or plan A, will need to be used in some instances. In addition, behaviorists may be more comfortable viewing EPP approaches as heavily focusing on antecedent management. Vice versa, as with other controversial issues in this section, proponents of EPP often overlook universal recommendations to use time-out as a singular strategy in the context of a positive reinforcement focused system. Similar to EPP's guidance on limit setting, time-out within BPT programs should be used sparingly. The two approaches differ in that BPT programs spend more time focusing on *how* to set limits. EPP supporters can also more accurately view behavioral approaches as tools for building skills and preventing future problems. As described previously, reinforcing effective emotion regulation, communication, and problem-solving strategies is actually encouraged as a primary focus of BPT strategies independently of how limits are enforced.

Even with a more accurate conceptualization of EPP programs, there are two main issues with EPP philosophy claims. First, there is little evidence indicating that positive approaches alone are sufficient to motivate children to behave appropriately (Larzelere et al., 2020). In fact, several studies have shown that positive parenting components alone are significantly less effective than programs that include both positive parenting and discipline components (e.g., including time-out; see Quetsch et al., 2015 for a review). Second, while research on two programs (CPT and TIK) is promising, there is not yet enough empirical support to recommend EPP approaches in the face of a vast literature supporting time-out and BPT.

In a final note on EPP, we are concerned that some programs advocate strategies that risk reinforcing undesirable behavior. While using positive parenting strategies (as encouraged by both EPP and BPT programs), caregiver behavior such as reasoning, negotiating, explaining, and using supportive touch may inadvertently reinforce problem behavior *when used during or immediately following inappropriate behavior*. Although CPS cautions caregivers against this "poor timing," other EPP approaches do not. Similarly, collaborative problem-solving approaches that use "taking a break" as a solution may reinforce escape in some circumstances. In summary, although the theory behind EPP approaches sounds appealing, professionals and caregivers are cautioned against using them in place of an empirically supported treatment (e.g., time-out, BPT) until more evidence is available.

> **Strategies that risk reinforcing undesirable behavior**

7.3.6   Is Time-Out Widely Unacceptable?

With the advent of the EPP movement, it seems plausible that disciplinary strategies like time-out have become widely unpopular and unacceptable. Internationally, parents and therapists have raised concerns that time-out is too demanding, too harsh, or will otherwise be perceived negatively (Norway, Bjørseth et al., 2010; New Zealand, Woodfield et al., 2020). For example, the Australian Association for Infant Mental Health Inc. has expressed concern that children, especially those under the age of 3, will not learn to regulate their feelings while in time-out (AAIMHI, 2016). Within the United States, Spanish-speaking Hispanic families and more recent Korean immigrants have reported using time-out less than those from other groups (Kim & Hong, 2007; Regalado et al., 2004).

Overall, however, acceptability research shows that time-out for child behavior management is a widely accepted practice. As described previously, the National Survey of Early Childhood Health (2000) revealed that 70% of all caregivers in the United States reported using time-out with children between the ages of 19–35 months (Regalado et al., 2004). Time-out is not only acceptable but recommended by a variety of professional organizations (American Academy of Pediatrics, AAP, 1998, 2018; Substance Abuse and Mental Health Services Administration, SAMHSA, 2011).

> **Time-out for child behavior management is a widely accepted practice**

Researchers have investigated time-out's acceptability. Taken together, this research shows that parents, children, and teachers typically rate time-out more positively than physical punishment, as moderately acceptable overall, and less positively than positive reinforcement strategies (Adams & Kelley, 1992; Blampied & Kahan, 1992; Dadds et al., 1987; Forcino et al., 2019; Jones et al., 1998; Passini et al., 2014). In addition, education and training has been shown to increase acceptability (Singh & Katz, 1985). For a review of time-out acceptability research, see Turner and Watson, 1999.

7.4 Legal Issues

Legal issues related to seclusion and restraint

Several legal issues relating to time-out have been raised. These largely involve the constructs of *seclusion* and *restraint*. Seclusion has been defined differently by governing bodies, but in general, it refers to involuntary confinement of an individual to a room alone in which they are physically prevented from leaving. In turn, restraint is defined as a method of involuntarily limiting an individual's freedom of physical movement. Restraint methods may include physical force (e.g., holding), mechanical devices (e.g., non-self-releasing lap belts), or chemical agents (e.g., sedative medications). Numerous organizations have produced guidelines indirectly limiting the use of time-out as delivered in clinical or educational settings by targeting seclusion and restraint (Joint Commission on Accreditation of Healthcare Organizations, 2009; US Department of Education, 2010). Protective guidelines provide important safeguards and have been born out of past cases of abuse and cruelty. These organizations are typically charged with ensuring the safety and ethical treatment of vulnerable populations, for example, children in schools, incapacitated older adults, individuals with severe mental illness, and incarcerated individuals.

Seclusion and restraint to be used sparingly and as last resort only

Within the legal documents, policies, and reports put forth by these institutions, long lists of legal definitions and rules for classifying circumstances abound. It is beyond the scope of this book to cover each policy in detail; however, in general, most policies indicate that seclusion and restraint should be used sparingly and as last resorts only when safety is at risk. Accordingly, some situations in which time-out is used seem to fit with these requirements. For instance, if time-out is being used as part of compliance training because a child has been running into traffic, some may consider this an issue of safety. Time-out could also be used to protect other students from an aggressive child in the classroom. Nonisolation methods of time-out are preferable, so using a time-out room as a back-up procedure seems to fit with the "last resort" guidelines.

Time-out components affected when seclusion and restraint are prohibited

Nevertheless, certain governing bodies do not allow any form of isolation or restraint in relation to time-out. This prohibits some therapists, teachers, childcare providers, and foster parents from using some components of time-out procedures. Common components affected are (1) carrying a child to a time-out location, (2) holding or putting the child back in the time-out location, and (3) using a time-out room as a back-up for escape. As such, schools, BPT programs, and social welfare agencies have published detailed clarifications of their disciplinary policies, even modifying them in many cases.

7.4.1 Modifications of Time-Out Procedures

Modifications Related to Seclusion

When governmental or institutional bodies prevent the standard 1-minute placement of a child in a back-up room for escape from the time-out chair, procedures have been modified. Some clinics use a half-door, also called a *Dutch door* or *pony door* so that the child is not completely separated from the rest of the room. Similarly, a baby gate or playpen may be used for smaller children. In other cases, especially foster care, a caregiver remains with the child in the back-up room so that the child is not left alone in a seclusion situation. Typically, the caregiver is coached to face and lean on the door frame to block escape, avoid giving attention, and protect themselves from aggression. Finally, if there are regulations against locking the back-up room, a door without a lock is used. If needed, an adult can block the door with their foot or by holding the doorknob for short periods. Regardless of modification to the back-up room, professionals must ensure that the space meets physical standards put forth by governing bodies (e.g., minimum size, light, ventilation).

Modifications Related to Restraint

In general, time-out procedures requiring an adult to hold the child in place are not recommended as they are more likely to increase attention and create physical power struggles. If regulations prevent carrying the child to time-out or repeatedly putting the child back in the chair, alternatives can be implemented. If the child refuses to go to or stay in the time-out location, a back-up procedure (e.g., back-up room, restriction of privilege, deferred time-out) can be used. Alternatively, reinforcing stimuli (e.g., toys, other children) can be removed from the immediate environment to "bring the time-out to the child." This is also called swoop and go in parent–child interaction therapy (see Chapter 8 for more details).

7.4.2 Conclusion

Modifications to time-out procedures may be necessary to ensure compliance with legal and regulatory guidelines in a variety of settings, particularly in foster care and school environments. It is important to check with agency, institutional, statewide, and national regulations before implementing specific time-out protocols. Imperative for legal and ethical reasons, legal guardians should be in agreement with selected time-out procedures. It is also critical to attend to potential experiences of seclusion and restraint. Above all, it is important that our treatment methods demonstrate respect for the rights of children, a vulnerable population.

Modifications may be legally necessary in some cases

7.5 Ethical Issues

Closely related to legal issues are ethical concerns regarding time-out. Professional organizations outline ethical guidelines for work with children in numerous fields. In some form or another, ethical codes guiding psychologists, medical providers, counselors, social workers, and educators require members to benefit individuals under their charge while limiting harm. The ethical codes of the American Psychological and American Counseling Associations term this *beneficence* and *nonmaleficence* (ACA, 2014; APA, 2017). Professional ethical guidelines for a variety of relevant fields herald respect for individuals' rights and dignity and providing competent care.

Ethical codes aim to benefit individuals while limiting harm

Psychologists and physicians must base care on available scientific knowledge (American Medical Association, 2016; APA, 2017) while counselors should use science or theory as a guide.

Accordingly, both champions and opponents of time-out have examined it as an ethical question. Time-outs' proponents cite its positive outcomes (e.g., improvements in child compliance, externalizing behavior problems, overall mental health) as ethical obligations to utilize it when appropriate. Based on the scientific literature, one could argue that withholding available evidence-based practices, such as time-out or BPT approaches that use it, is unethical.

On the other hand, critics have cited theoretical arguments that time-out's negative effects outweigh its utility. According to ethical guidelines, it is important to weigh the benefits and risks of individual treatments. As psychologists, we weigh the scientific evidence. While time-out may be challenging to administer in certain situations and produce a temporary extinction burst, according to the literature, its effects are greatly beneficial, and there are no known negative long-term impacts. Measures should be taken, however, to minimize immediate distress for families using time-out. For example, in addressing issues with conducting time-out with children exhibiting symptoms of autism or developmental delays, strategies have been developed to ease into time-out to decrease the extinction burst. Described as a *readiness phase*, McNeil and colleagues have suggested the possibility of spending a few sessions using a hand-over-hand guide for the consequence for noncompliance during parent–child interaction therapy compliance training to prepare both the caregiver and the child with special needs for the time-out phase (McNeil et al., 2018). Ultimately, looking to research is important to determine the most efficient (i.e., maximum benefit, minimum distress) method of treatment. For time-out, this may mean using the least restrictive environment, shortest duration, and most consistent administration known to be effective for the specific individual and target behavior.

7.6   Conclusion

Deciding to use time-out, or any other parenting approach for that matter, can be a complex issue. There are many factors to consider related to time-out, punishment, or behavioral approaches as a whole. Based on our review of the literature, frequently cited concerns with time-out related to trauma, physiological harm, or otherwise negative long-term effects have no research to support them. While time-out and behavioral parenting approaches are not the only effective treatments for child behavior management, they are some of the most empirically validated. Despite controversial theories, within an overall positive approach to parenting, time-out has a proven track record of effectively managing child behavior problems.

8

Parent–Child Interaction Therapy (PCIT) Time-Out as an Exemplar

In this chapter, we review the time-out procedure prescribed in the parent–child interaction therapy (PCIT) program as an exemplar. First, we explain the basic components of PCIT. Next, we describe the specific steps of time-out used in PCIT as well as key considerations for therapists in teaching time-out to families. Finally, we touch on the time-out procedure within the context of the entire program.

PCIT, first developed as an intervention for children with disruptive behavior problems, ages 2 to 7 years, is an evidence-based treatment for a variety of behavior problems, worldwide. For more information, see the *PCIT Protocol* (Eyberg & Funderburk, 2011) and parent–child interaction therapy (McNeil & Hembree-Kigin, 2010). PCIT has been adapted for use with children younger than 2 and older than 7 years. For modifications to discipline strategies for younger and older children, see Chapter 3.

As briefly described in Chapter 5 of this book, PCIT involves two phases: child-directed interaction (CDI) and parent-directed interaction (PDI). During CDI, caregivers learn and practice a variety of positive parenting skills to reinforce the child's desirable behavior. Chief among these are the PRIDE skills, which include praise, reflection, imitation, description, and enjoyment. Caregivers spend 5 minutes per day using these skills in one-on-one playtime with their child. In addition, caregivers learn to avoid asking questions, giving commands, and using criticism during practice sessions, to keep the child in the lead. The goal of CDI is to improve the caregiver–child relationship and establish interactions with the caregiver, or "time-in," as reinforcing. In PCIT, caregivers must demonstrate competency in the CDI skills before beginning with PDI skills or any work with time-out.

PCIT involves two phases

Time-in during PCIT

8.1 Introducing Time-Out

Before proceeding with teaching any new discipline strategy, therapists should review previously used discipline strategies with families, particularly identifying issues related to culture, values, and abilities. Negative experiences with time-out including ineffectiveness, difficulty implementing, and trauma histories should be discussed. Alternatives for caregivers or children whose physical characteristics or strong personal objections preclude carrying out a standard time-out can be found in Section 8.5 of this chapter and in Chapter 3. For families who have simply found time-out to be too effortful or ineffective in the past, therapists are encouraged to describe the time-out in PCIT as unique and "therapeutic," given its focus on extreme consistency, predictability, and structure. Families can be asked about their willingness to "experiment" with this new version of time-out to see if its high level of structure will work for their child. For families with anxiety or trauma histories, the consistency and predictability of time-out can also be reassuring. Clinicians may discuss the fact that time-out should be delivered in a calm and controlled fashion. The goal is for caregivers to employ emotion regulation strategies when implementing time-out. In this way, a positive discipline approach can replace anger-based, punishment strategies such as yelling, delivering harsh consequences, and spanking. Therapists can assure families that there is no evidence that time-out traumatizes or re-traumatizes children. In fact, research shows that PCIT can actually reduce trauma symptoms in children. For more background, see Chapters 2 and 7.

8.2 PDI Teach Session

In PCIT, the strategies, rules, and procedures for discipline and time-out are typically taught to caregivers only (i.e., no children) in a 1-hour "PDI Teach." This session follows the caregivers' achievement of proficiency in the CDI skills within the CDI phase of treatment and prior to any discipline or time-out coaching or implementation in the PDI phase of treatment.

8.2.1 Effective Commands

During the PDI Teach session, caregivers learn about giving effective commands to improve child compliance. Briefly, effective commands are: (1) direct (told) rather than indirect (asked), (2) positively stated, (3) given one at a time, (4) specific rather than vague, (5) age-appropriate, (6) stated politely and respectfully, (7) explained before they are given or after they are obeyed, and (8) used only when necessary. Please, see Appendix 2 for examples of how to make less effective commands more effective. In PCIT, time-out is introduced as a consequence for noncompliance to direct commands only. This way, caregivers can control when they use commands and consequently when they may need to implement time-out. Once caregivers and children can follow the time-out procedure with integrity, time-out is generalized to other types of target behavior.

8.2.2 Effective Follow-Through

Praising child compliance

Effective commands are taught in conjunction with effective follow-through. See Appendix 3 for a concise visual summary of correct follow-through (Thanks to the WVU PCIT Lab and Erinn Victory for assistance with developing the images for these diagrams). If the child complies with a command, he or she receives a labeled (i.e., specific) praise (e.g., **"Thank you for following** directions.") and other positive social reinforcement through continued time-in. If the child does not comply within 5 seconds, the caregiver is trained to give a verbatim chair warning statement, **"If you don't (insert original command), you'll have to sit on the time-out chair."** The child then has 5 more seconds to comply. Compliance is met with a labeled praise and return to the use of positive parenting skills for time-in. Noncompliance is followed with another verbatim statement: **"You didn't do what I told you to do, so you have to sit on the time-out chair."** The following time-out procedure is explained to caregivers during the PDI Teach session, and handouts are provided.

Time-out chair warning for noncompliance

Chair Time-Out

When a time-out is warranted, the caregiver should gently lift the child from behind with arms clasped under the child's armpits and across the chest in a barrel hold. The caregiver is to quickly and gently remove any objects from the child's fingers before carrying him or her to the chair. Next, the caregiver should place the child's bottom on the chair and step away from "the kicking zone," so the child cannot kick, hit, or grab them. The caregiver is told to say, **"Stay on the chair until I say you can get off."** Then the caregiver should engage in another activity within eyesight of the child. Ideally, the activity is to appear to be enjoyable to the child (e.g., playing with toys), so the child will be motivated to finish with time-out as soon as possible. The caregiver is taught to watch the child out of the corner of their eye without providing attention through direct eye contact. The caregiver should not provide any attention, especially speaking to or touching the child during time-out. The caregiver is to time for 3 minutes and then listen for 5 seconds of silence from the child.

The child must stay on the time-out chair for 3 minutes + 5 seconds of silence

Ending Time-Out

After the child has completed 3 minutes in the chair and remained quiet for 5 seconds at the end, the caregiver should approach the chair. While standing out of the "kicking zone," the caregiver is told to say, **"You are sitting quietly on the chair."** This is meant to reinforce quiet behavior on the chair in the future. Then the caregiver should ask, **"Are you ready to [insert original command]?"** If the child agrees or makes efforts to comply, the caregiver should accompany the child to ensure the task is completed. However, if the child says, "No" or refuses, the caregiver is to restart time-out, again saying, **"Stay on the chair until I say you can get off."** The child must again sit on the chair for 3 minutes plus 5 seconds of quiet before the caregiver approaches and repeats the statements above. This continues until the child complies with the original instruction. In this way, the child cannot use time-out to escape demands. When the child complies with the original instruction, the caregiver must give a neutral comment, such as, "okay" or "thank you." This will prevent the reinforcement of the chain of behavior that necessitated time-out to motivate compliance.

Compliance with original command

Although the child has complied with the original command, the time-out procedure will not yet be complete. To enhance learning, the caregiver must immediately give a simple follow-up command to establish compliance. For example, if the original command was, "Come to the table," the caregiver

Follow-up command

could add a follow-up command, such as "Now, put your napkin on your lap." If the child does not comply, the caregiver must return to the chair warning statement. If the child complies within 5 seconds after the follow-up command or after the chair warning statement, the caregiver should give an enthusiastic, labeled praise for listening the first time. This will end the time-out procedure. If the child does not comply after the chair warning statement, the caregiver must return to following the steps of the chair time-out above. In other words, the only way a child can be finished with time-out is by sitting on the chair for 3 minutes, remaining quiet for at least 5 seconds, complying with the original command, and complying with the follow-up command.

Rules While on the Time-Out Chair

During the PDI Teach session, caregivers learn the following rules regarding acceptable behavior during a PCIT chair time-out. It is permissible for the child to make noise (e.g., scream, make negative statements) and move around on the chair (e.g., gesture, kick, turn around). Attempting to control these behaviors will only reinforce them with attention. However, scooting, rocking, standing on the chair, or putting more than 50% of the child's weight off of the chair is not permitted. These behaviors are either safety risks or provide escape from the boredom of time-out. For example, a child could fall while tipping the chair or gain access to a fun activity (e.g., grab a toy, start kicking the wall) by scooting the chair to another location. The first time a child engages in one of these unacceptable behaviors during time-out, the caregiver is instructed to administer the *once in a lifetime warning* which states: **"You got off the chair before I said you could. If you get off the chair again, you will go to the time-out room."** If, after this warning, the child breaks one of the time-out rules again, even if it is during a future time-out, the warning is not given again.

Once in a lifetime time-out room warning

Handling Escape From the Chair

Caregivers are taught the following procedure for responding to a violation of the time-out chair rules. If the child violates a chair rule after the *once in a lifetime warning* has been given, the caregiver should state, **"You got off the chair before I said you could, so you have to go to the time-out room."** At the same time, the caregiver is to quickly and gently pick the child up from behind in a barrel hold and carry him or her to the back-up space. No other talking to the child is permitted. The caregiver should set the child down gently on his or her bottom as far away from the door into the room as possible. Then the caregiver must leave the room swiftly, and close the door without pinching the child's fingers. The caregiver should then hold the door closed while standing within the child's line of sight but without providing direct eye contact for 1 minute. After 1 minute, the caregiver must listen for 5 seconds of silence from the child. When this is achieved, without talking, the caregiver is to enter the room, carefully pick up the child as before, and return the child to the time-out chair. Immediately after, the caregiver should step away and repeat the phrase, **"Stay on the chair until I say you can get off."**

The child stays in the back-up space for 1 minute + 5 seconds of silence

8.2.3 Return to Child-Directed Interaction

Following successful completion of the time-out procedure, caregivers are encouraged to return to CDI or PRIDE skills. These skills emphasize the reinforcing nature of positive caregiver–child interactions available outside of time-out, while returning the child to the lead. The child may be upset or avoid the caregiver immediately after time-out, but most young children quickly recover and can be redirected with CDI skills. Caregivers should re-establish calm, positive interactions for at least several minutes before issuing any further directives. A ratio of many more positive interactions to negative interactions is vital in a warm caregiver–child relationship. In turn this relationship is crucial for ensuring a child's desire to please his or her caregiver. The return to positive interactions with the caregiver sends an important message to the child that the caregiver found the noncompliant behavior to be unacceptable but still loves and enjoys the child.

8.2.4 Planning for At-Home Practice

During the PDI Teach session, clinicians should discuss with families the time-out spaces they will use at home. Although the family will not practice PDI procedures outside of clinic until after the first PDI coaching session, it is useful to share important considerations ahead of time. First, the family should identify a sturdy, adult-sized chair, preferably without arms, and a location in the home where it can be placed away from walls and anything else a child could reach while sitting in it. The chair can be used for other purposes throughout the day but should be near the appropriate location for time-out. Similarly, the chair and selected location should be close enough to where the non-compliance is most likely to occur in the home, so the caregiver can easily guide the child to time-out when warranted. The best time-out chair location is away from interesting activities (e.g., out of view of television) but within sight of the caregiver for supervision.

Second, the space the family plans to use as a back-up for violation of the time-out chair rules at home must be selected. The space should be enclosed, well-lit, appropriately sized (at least 5 feet by 5 feet; Eyberg & Funderburk, 2011), and safe. Many families identify the child's bedroom. This can work well. As with the clinic space, caregivers should make adjustments to the room to increase safety and decrease stimulation. It is important to talk through potential pitfalls with families in advance. For instance, is there any furniture the child could tip over or jump off of? Some caregivers worry that using the child's bedroom for time-out may create negative associations with the space. In our clinical experiences, this has not been a problem. To mitigate these worries, families can increase the use of the child's bedroom for positive activities throughout the day (e.g., reading stories, playing games together). Other families prefer to use a parent's bedroom because it has fewer toys to remove. Families should be cautioned against using bathrooms. Children can get into medications and cleaners or have lots of fun splashing water, creating messes, and slipping hazards. Caregivers should also be discouraged from using closets as they tend to be dark, small spaces.

8.2.5 Planning for the First Discipline Coaching Session

Once the basic procedures have been explained, families should be mentally and physically prepared before their first discipline coaching session. The first therapeutic time-out procedures in clinic and at home can be mentally and physically exhausting for both caregivers and children. This should be made clear to families in advance. First, physical abilities should be established. Clinicians must discuss with each caregiver, his or her capacity and willingness to carry the child to the time-out chair and back-up space repeatedly if necessary. Alternatives can be arranged if this is not feasible; see older child protocol in Chapter 3. Next, setting events should be addressed. Clinicians should obtain a caregiver's assurance that the child will be well-fed, well-rested, and will have used the toilet (if appropriate) before the first discipline session. This will decrease risks of extreme emotion dysregulation, toileting accidents, and escape in the form of trips to the bathroom. The family and therapist's schedules following the first discipline session should be cleared in case multiple chair time-outs and trips to the back-up space are required. It is important that the child does not escape caregiver demands because the family or clinician "runs out of time" as this may further reinforce noncompliance, tantrums, and aggression. The therapist may explain to the caregiver that it is considered beneficial to have a time-out during the first session, because caregivers and the child will learn a great deal by practicing the time-out procedures under the close supervision and coaching of a trained therapist.

8.3 First PDI Coaching Session

8.3.1 Preparing the Room

Safety precautions

In preparation for a PDI coaching session in the clinic, the therapy room should be stripped of all unnecessary materials and potential safety risks. Clinicians should imagine how a child seeking attention or escape may use materials in the room to achieve these goals and how the environment could interfere with the caregiver's effective implementation of time-out. Common steps include installing child-safe power outlet covers, removing or securing shelving units that can be tipped over, locking cabinets, taking art, blinds, and curtains off the walls, removing furniture that children may climb on, and taking all but a handful of small toys out of the room. Toys may become projectiles or tripping hazards for caregivers when carrying the child to time-out. Other more intensive precautions may be taken, such as installing unbreakable glass windows and mirrors, moving light switches to the outside of the room, updating doors handles and latches to prevent fingers being pinched, and making sure no sinks or hand soap/sanitizer dispensers are in the room (e.g., medical settings). Finally, a sturdy, adult-sized chair, preferably without arms, should be placed away from walls and anything else a child could reach while sitting in it.

8.3.2 Preparing the Back-Up Space

In clinic, the time-out back-up space is often connected to the room where the time-out chair is located. The room should be comfortable, safe, and as boring as possible. The back-up space must be well-lit and large enough that the child is comfortable (at least 16 square feet). As with the main room where PDI is being conducted, potentially dangerous items should be removed. In addition, no toys should be available in the back-up room. The back-up room door should have a window or opening allowing the child to see that their caregiver is nearby. Some agencies or children (e.g., those in foster care) may have specific rules about being left in a room alone, even for 1 minute. To accommodate this, some clinics use a half door or "pony" door for their back-up space. Clinicians should assess the risks of children climbing over these doors in advance.

8.3.3 Beginning the First Discipline Coaching Session

Once caregivers' willingness to participate in the first discipline session and all logistical details have been addressed, many caregivers benefit from a "pep talk." In this pep talk, caregivers should be warned that the first discipline session is often longer and more demanding than any other session or time-out. During the first time-out, many oppositional and defiant children test their caregivers' limits, limits which have likely proven to be flexible in the past. It may be helpful to obtain a verbal commitment from caregivers that they are willing to "go the distance," or not give up, until the child has successfully completed the time-out procedure. Clinicians can reassure caregivers that they will be coached and supported every second of the first discipline session.

Pep talk for caregivers

8.3.4 Teaching PDI to the Child

At all coaching sessions, children are included. At the start of this first PDI coaching session, caregivers are coached to explain and role-play with their child how to "listen" (i.e., following direct commands) and what will happen if they choose not to listen (i.e., demonstrating each permutation of the time-out procedure). Role-play can involve using a stuffed animal (e.g., "Mr. Bear") who is "learning to listen." Each rule of the time-out chair should be explained to the child in some way. In our clinical experience, children are more likely to end up in time-out during the first session if their caregiver is coached through teaching them about time-out, rather than if the therapist teaches time-out directly to the child.

8.3.5 Coaching PDI

In all PDI coaching sessions, caregivers are coached to engage in a short period of CDI-only skills practice followed by a longer period of PDI skills practice with their child. To start, PDI skills practice focuses on coaching caregivers to give effective "play commands" with effective follow-through. Play commands are intended to have a high probability of success. "Hand me…" commands, such as, "Hand me that blue crayon" are popular. In the first PDI coaching session, caregivers can introduce the change by saying, **"Now it's my turn to choose what we play, and we're going to practice listening and minding. If you mind me quickly, we'll have lots more time to play together."** One play command should be given intermittently for every 1 minute of CDI skills. Warning statements, chair time-outs, and back-up space procedures are coached for noncompliance according to protocol.

Throughout the PDI phase of treatment, caregivers are assigned daily PDI practice homework in addition to the established 5 minutes of daily CDI skills practice homework. As families complete daily homework consistently and demonstrate proficiency in PDI skills in session, homework and coaching gradually advance to include more realistic commands and situations.

8.4 Gradual Roll-Out Approach

As described previously, in PCIT, time-out is first used only for noncompliance to direct commands. To set families up for success, PCIT uses a gradual process for introducing effective commands and time-out at home. This competency-based progression is intended to shape caregivers' and children's behavior to minimize distress and errors while optimizing skill acquisition. A brief summary of steps can be viewed in the diagram in Figure 1 (Thanks to Nancy Wallace and the West Virginia University PCIT Lab for assistance with formatting the staircase). In PCIT, families usually practice the commands on

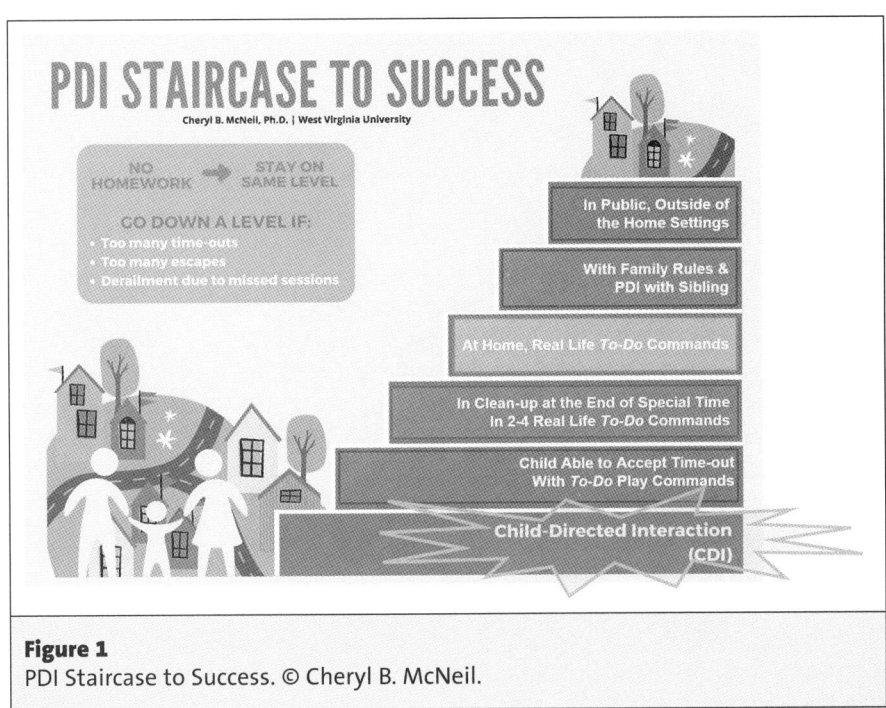

Figure 1
PDI Staircase to Success. © Cheryl B. McNeil.

each step of the staircase for at least one session and for one week at home before progressing. For more details, refer to the PCIT Protocol (Eyberg & Funderburk, 2011).

8.4.1 Time-Out for Other Behavior

Once time-out is effective for noncompliance throughout the day at home, time-out can be generalized as a consequence for other types of undesirable behavior. Many families choose to establish a "house rule." An appropriate house rule targets misbehavior that occurs at least daily (if not many times per day) and that is *never* acceptable. "No hurting" is a popular house rule which can encompass hitting, kicking, biting, pushing, etc. Only one or two house rules should be active at once. Otherwise, the child may have too many time-outs, leading to parent–child conflict and decreased compliance. Caregivers can introduce a house rule by labeling the target behavior for a few days to one week before implementing. If a child hits at home, the caregiver may say, "You hit your brother. Remember the no hurting rule. If you hit next week, it will be an automatic time-out." Following implementation of the rule, caregivers simply label the violation and take the child directly to time-out. The same time-out procedure is followed except that compliance to a command is not required to end time-out. Instead, a caregiver simply states, **"You are sitting quietly on the chair. Remember we don't (insert house rule)."**

Establishing a house rule

By gradually introducing time-out for compliance and then a maximum of one or two house rules, expectations for child behavior are reasonable, and the family is set up for success. This structure limits the chances that caregivers will abruptly send the child to time-out for vague misbehavior. The child always has a choice, provided through the warning statement for noncompliance, or has been prepared in advance through the introduction of the house rule.

8.5 Alternatives to Chairs, Back-Up Spaces, and Carrying Children

The standard PCIT time-out procedure is not always suited for the unique needs of all families and settings. For situations in which carrying a child is not feasible, the swoop and go procedure may be used. In this approach, rather than bring the child to time-out, caregivers bring time-out to the child. Using the swoop and go procedure, if a child escapes from the chair, an alternative *once in a lifetime warning* is given: **"You got off the chair before I said you could. If you get off the chair again, I will take the toys and wait outside the room."** If the child does not comply, the following statement is made, **"You got off the chair before I said you could, so I will take the toys and wait outside the room."** The caregiver then quickly removes all toys and reinforcers, including themselves, from the room for 1 minute plus 5 seconds of silence. The procedure is less effective if not all sources of reinforcement can be removed (e.g., a room full of toys). The swoop and go procedure

Swoop and go procedure

eliminates the need to get the child to stay on a chair and thus the use of a back-up room.

8.6 Conclusion

The PCIT time-out is just one example of how time-out elements can be combined for the effective management of child behavior problems. However, this particular formulation has demonstrated consistent effectiveness across thousands of families (Eyberg et al., 2008). We hope that this structure is educational in helping families learn to engage in safe, consistent discipline strategies. In the following chapter, this structure is loosely followed with tailoring and modifications in a case study.

9

Case Vignette

To protect the confidentiality of clients, this case study uses fictional names and represents a merging of details from several actual cases.

9.1 Case Background

Eliana was a 6-year-old girl brought to clinic by her parents, Marcos "Papi" (age 29) and Luis "Pá" (age 30). The family sought help managing Eliana's emotional outbursts. Marcos reported that about 2 to 3 times on a typical school night, and up to 10 times on an average Saturday, Eliana experienced tantrums. These were typically in response to not getting something she wanted (e.g., ice cream) or being asked to engage in a nonpreferred task (e.g., get in the bathtub). Tantrums lasted from 2 to 30 minutes and included whining, screaming, crying, name calling, hitting, pinching, throwing objects at her parents, and breaking toys. Regarding compliance, Eliana's parents reported that, when given 10 simple instructions to follow throughout the day (e.g., go get your coat, hand me the cup), she would initially comply with 0 or 1 of them. When allowed to engage in preferred activities, Eliana was described as an outgoing, smart, and sweet child. She had no history of medical problems, developmental delays, or other special needs. *[Behavior problems at home]*

Eliana started kindergarten a few months before her intake. She also had tantrums at school, but these were less frequent and shorter-lived than at home. Teachers explained that Eliana sometimes yelled or hid under her desk when she did not want to participate in an activity, but this usually stopped after 1 or 2 minutes. Noncompliance and tantrums were more frequent at the beginning of the school year. Eliana had responded well to a classroom-based positive behavior incentive program. Students could earn special privileges like being line-leader or choosing a prize out of a box for good behavior. Similarly, her social behavior had improved somewhat since the start of the year. Still, Eliana sometimes yelled or took things from peers when her classmates had a toy she wanted or didn't want to play according to her rules. On one occasion, Eliana's parents were called to school when she pushed another child off the swing she wanted to use on the playground, resulting in a minor injury. *[Behavior problems in school]*

Eliana's parents described an increased level of parenting and marital stress due to her behavior. They could not relax and enjoy family time because they felt they had to "walk on eggshells" to avoid tantrums. The family avoided bringing Eliana on outings to restaurants, stores, and the zoo because they were embarrassed by her outbursts. In addition, her parents disagreed on how *[Resulting parenting and marital stress]* to manage Eliana's tantrums. Luis pointed out that his parents had "popped" him when he "got out of line" as a child, and he believed strongly that this method had helped him learn how to behave. Therefore, Luis explained that he spanked Eliana with an open hand on the bottom if she tried to hit either parent. According to Luis, the spankings caused Eliana to avoid any physical aggression toward either parent when Luis was present. However, Eliana still hit and pinched Marcos when Luis was at work. Marcos did not report these incidents to Luis because he did not want Eliana to be spanked. Marcos had also been raised in a home where his father used physical discipline, sometimes striking the children with a belt. His mother had yelled at the children frequently and threatened to tell his father if they misbehaved. He remembered being afraid of his father as a young boy and experienced high levels of anxiety as an adult. Marcos wanted to develop a more supportive, nurturing relationship between Eliana and her parents than he had growing up. He and Luis had agreed not to use physical discipline before Eliana was born. Over the past 2 years, Luis had decided that spanking was one of the only effective strategies to manage Eliana's aggressive behavior. Luis and Marcos often had arguments about how to discipline Eliana.

Baseline behavior management strategies

Both parents reported trying numerous strategies to decrease tantrums and noncompliance. They had tried speaking calmly and holding Eliana when she was upset, talking to her about the importance of respecting her parents, taking away electronics for misbehavior, sending her to her room until she calmed down, and even time-out. Marcos described the following time-out procedure: If Eliana refused to follow directions or hit her father, she would be told to stand in a corner for time-out. This often increased the intensity of the tantrum, and Marcos sometimes had to chase Eliana around the house and guide her to the corner by the hand. While in time-out, Eliana usually screamed at her father and made hurtful statements like, "You're mean!", "I want Grandma.", and "I hate you." She also banged her hands and kicked the walls. Marcos explained that he had to stand near Eliana to prevent her from leaving the corner, damaging the wall, or yelling. Time-outs lasted until Elaina was "calm," which could be up to 20 or 30 minutes on a "bad day." Both parents admitted that time-out was exhausting and "did not work" to improve behavior. Marcos reported feeling guilty for putting Eliana in time-out because he worried that it damaged their relationship. For these reasons, the family had not used time-out for the past 2 years. Lately, Eliana had been sent to her room for misbehavior until she calmed down. Her parents noted that Eliana had broken some of her toys while in her room and snuck out of the room if parents were not waiting right outside to send her back immediately.

Cultural and family variables

The family noted the following cultural and family variables. Both parents had grown up attending Catholic church but currently did not identify as religious. Both Luis and Marcos could trace their lineage back to Mexico and still had some extended family members living there. They spoke both Spanish and English in the home. Both parents worked full time outside of the home; Marcos worked days, and Luis worked from late afternoon through midnight. Eliana was an only child. Her parents had undergone a long and expensive process of conceiving Eliana using a surrogate. Eliana had a close relationship with Marcos' mother, "Abue," who lived nearby. Her grandmother spoke Spanish in the home but could speak English as well. Eliana spent Friday nights at her grandmother's home nearly every week. Eliana's grandmother enjoyed "spoiling" Eliana with treats and privileges. She reported good behavior from Eliana for the most part, except when her parents came to pick her up after a visit.

9.2 Treatment Plan and Goals

The family agreed to participate in a short-term, problem-focused family therapy model. They listed reducing tantrums and aggression and improving compliance as their top goals for treatment. Luis and Marcos stated their commitment to attending 1-hour, weekly appointments with Eliana for an estimated 6–10 sessions. They were encouraged to include extended family members in appointments as well if possible. Marcos expressed interest in having his mother attend. Eliana's parents were introduced to the idea that Eliana could benefit more if her parents learned behavior management and play therapy skills for daily use than if she simply visited her own individual therapist for a short time each week. They understood that their active participation and weekly skills practice at home would be a vital part of therapy.

9.2.1 Treatment Session 1 (Relationship-Building Didactic & Coaching)

Treatment began with psychoeducation for caregivers. Eliana, her parents, and her grandmother attended. Luis and Marcos learned basic behavioral principles such as reinforcement for positive behavior and differential attention, while Eliana's grandmother listened and played with her on the floor. The idea of child-led play was also introduced (Eyberg & Funderburk, 2011). This 5-minute, daily, 1-on-1 play session with each parent would be a time for Eliana to "be in charge," allowing her to lead the play in a preferred activity while having no demands placed on her. Marcos liked this idea and believed that Eliana would be more likely to listen to him if their relationship was stronger.

Introduction to behavior therapy

Luis expressed skepticism. He had hoped to increase behavioral expectations for Eliana and had difficulty accepting that playing with Eliana would improve her respect for authority. He explained that he had never played with Eliana before. These concerns were validated. Luis agreed to experiment by trying out "special playtime" for a week, however, and report any behavioral changes at the next session. Eliana's grandmother expressed understanding of content but seemed reticent to express her opinions. Eliana's family received handouts (in English and Spanish) and brief explanations about each of the PRIDE skills (i.e., praise, reflect, imitate, describe, enjoy) as well as the "Don't Skills" (i.e., questions, commands, and criticism; Eyberg & Funderburk, 2011). The therapist modeled each skill and had each caregiver take turns using them in role-plays. Eliana frequently interrupted during the didactic portion of the session, climbing on her Papi's lap, pulling his arm, and whining for him to come play with her.

Modeling and role play

PRIDE skills coaching

Finally, each parent was coached to use the skills in independent play with Eliana for a few minutes each. Luis caught on quickly to praising, imitating, and describing but demonstrated some resistance to using enthusiasm and imitation. Marcos's strongest skills were praising, imitating, and enjoyment. Both parents used many questions throughout child-led play. Eliana's parents each planned to engage in "special playtime" once per day with Eliana at home over the next week. Eliana's grandmother declined to be coached, but she agreed to practice the playtime at her house. Parents discussed appropriate locations, activities, and times of day for practice and received a tracking sheet to record daily practice.

9.2.2 Treatment Session 2 (Relationship-Building Coaching & Differential Attention)

The following week, only Marcos and his mother accompanied Eliana to the session. Marcos reported that it was not possible for both parents to take off work each week for therapy, and they preferred late afternoon appointments so as not to take Eliana out of school if possible. Therefore, Marcos planned to attend the appointment weekly with his mother and Eliana, since he could come after work. He would explain what was learned to Luis at home. Luis intended to continue implementing strategies at home and could attend Eliana's appointment on occasion if necessary. He was encouraged to call the therapist with any questions throughout treatment.

Reinforcing at-home practice tracking

Marcos had left his practice log at home. The therapist provided a blank copy on which Marcos filled in data indicating that he had practiced with Eliana on 5 of the past 7 days. Luis had practiced with Eliana on 2 days. It had been difficult for Luis to practice because he was at work during the afternoon and evening hours on weekdays. Eliana had enjoyed the playtime, but she was bossy and argumentative during play. She also had difficulty accepting that playtime was over after each session.

Coding child-directed interaction (CDI) skills

The therapist coded Marcos in child-led play with Eliana for 5 minutes. His mother again declined participation but listened and observed. Marcos used 2 specific praises (e.g., "I like your picture."), 4 reflections, 5 descriptions, 15 questions, 0 commands, and 0 negative comments. Marcos used excellent enthusiasm but tended to sit and watch rather than join in the play. Next, Marcos was coached in child-directed interaction (CDI) skills. He was extremely responsive to coaching. Marcos easily adjusted vague praises (e.g., "Good job!") to labeled praises like "Good job coloring inside the lines." He often chose to use emotional words in his praises (e.g., "I am proud of the way you…", "It makes me happy when…"). Marcos quickly picked up on ensuring reflections were phrased as statements (e.g., Eliana: "That's how you do it."; Marcos: "That *is* how you do it.") rather than questions (e.g., Eliana: "That's how you do it."; Marcos: "That's how you do it?"). Because he picked up on the basic CDI skills so quickly, he was also coached in two higher level skills: praising target behavior related to treatment goals and differential attention.

During a break from coaching, Marcos was prompted to complete a handout with the therapist about praising positive opposites. The therapist explained the concept of identifying desirable behavior that was incompatible with Eliana's problem behavior. The therapist provided examples before asking Marcos to identify some positive opposites. Marcos named "staying calm" as the opposite of throwing a tantrum, "using nice hands" as the opposite of hitting, "being quiet" as the opposite of yelling, and "sharing" as the opposite of taking toys from others. During the remaining coaching time, Marcos was coached to prioritize praising these positive opposites. Marcos did an outstanding job of praising Eliana several times for being quiet and using nice hands.

Finally, the therapist coached Marcos in providing differential attention for Eliana's annoying or obnoxious behavior. When Eliana took a toy from her father without asking, criticized her father's play, or grunted at her father in disapproval, Marcos was coached to ignore the behavior. He then drew attention to his own play using enthusiasm and describing. Finally, Marcos was coached to quickly praise the opposite of the negative behavior as soon as it stopped (e.g., "I like it when you let me have a turn."; "Thanks for letting me play my way."). Marcos' progress with differential attention was evident at the end of session when Eliana began arguing about leaving clinic. Without being coached, Marcos began talking aloud to himself about what the family would have for dinner, responding to Eliana's negative comments with neither eye contact nor discussion. Eliana was easily redirected after about 30 seconds and praised for getting calm.

Coaching differential attention

Again, the family was asked to practice their CDI skills with Eliana for 5 minutes daily with each caregiver and return the data sheet. In addition, they were encouraged to look for opportunities to praise the positive opposites and use differential social attention throughout the day.

9.2.3 Treatment Session 3 (Relationship-Building Coaching & Discipline Didactic)

It had been 2 weeks since Eliana's last therapy session. Marcos had cancelled her appointment the week before due to illness. He attended with Eliana alone, as his mother was now ill. Marcos returned a homework sheet indicating practice for 10 of the past 14 days (4 of which Eliana was ill). He explained that Luis had practiced with Eliana on weekends but had not documented it. Eliana's grandmother had practiced when Eliana stayed at her house as well. Eliana had responded well to differential attention following special playtime and no longer argued when her father started to clean up the toys. However, she still had several tantrums per day which often included physical aggression toward her Papi when her Pá was at work.

Marcos was coached briefly in CDI with Eliana. He demonstrated marked improvement in making praises specific, avoiding turning reflections into questions, and using differential attention for undesirable behavior. Marcos spontaneously praised Eliana for using a quiet voice and playing nicely with him. Coaching focused on helping Marcos imitate Eliana's play. Marcos admitted that he usually "stayed out of Eliana's way" during play because she quickly got frustrated with the way her father interfered. At first, when he began to engage with the toys, Eliana criticized him and knocked over his toys. After being coached to ignore, redirect, and praise the opposite behavior (e.g., "I like it when you let me build my tower tall."), these problems decreased.

Shaping positive social skills

Overall, Eliana and her father were observed smiling, laughing, and sharing positive touches much more often than at previous sessions. Marcos explained that his relationship with Eliana felt stronger, and they enjoyed spending time together more than they had just a few weeks ago.

Introducing time-out

Because Marcos had picked up the skills so quickly and had been practicing diligently at home, the PDI portion or discipline phase of treatment was introduced. Marcos received psychoeducation about the eight rules of effective commands (Eyberg & Funderburk, 2011), while Eliana played independently with toys. Since there was not enough time remaining in the session to teach the entire time-out procedure, the *big ignore* for noncompliance was introduced (McNeil & Hembree-Kigin, 2010). Using this strategy, if a child does not comply with direct instruction, the caregiver turns away and ignores their behavior for 45 seconds. The therapist explained and modeled this for Marcos.

The therapist then discussed using a structured command sequence. This consisted of giving an effective, direct instruction (e.g., "Hand me the doll."), waiting 5 seconds for compliance, issuing a warning for noncompliance (e.g., "If you don't hand me the doll, I will turn and ignore."), waiting 5 more seconds for compliance, and making the following statement for noncompliance ("You did not do what I told you, so I will turn and ignore.") followed by a 45-second big ignore. If at any time before the consequence statement was given, Eliana complied, the caregiver was instructed to provide labeled praise. Marcos expressed concern that Eliana was able to "get out of" listening and would not mind if he ignored her for 45 seconds. The therapist agreed with Marcos and reassured him that ignoring would simply serve as a placeholder for a more effective consequence to be introduced next session. This way, Eliana and her caregivers could acclimate to the command sequence gradually. This way, the family would have time to practice time-out in session next week before trying it out on their own. It was recommended that Luis also attend the next session to learn the procedure firsthand.

Marcos was coached briefly in giving several simple play commands with Eliana while using CDI skills (e.g., "Hand me a blue crayon."). The commands were introduced with the statement, "It's time to practice listening." Eliana was 100% compliant, so the two were later coached to role-play the big ignore for noncompliance. The family's homework was to continue with special playtime for 5 minutes daily, during which they would give 3 play commands. The command sequence, including labeled praise for compliance or big ignore for noncompliance, was to be used with these play commands only. Eliana's father was encouraged to discipline Eliana as he normally would at other times for now.

9.2.4 Treatment Session 4 (Compliance Training & Time-Out Coaching)

Before this session the therapist and family planned to be available for up to an hour after the appointment. The family understood the potential for this session to be longer. Eliana, her parents, and grandmother attended. They brought homework sheets indicating practice of both special playtime and listening practice for 7 of the past 7 days, with Marcos practicing on weekdays and Luis practicing on weekends. Eliana was 100% compliant with commands on 5 of the 7 days. On two of the days, she did not comply with a command to put a toy away, so her parent followed the command sequence including the big ignore. Eliana did not seem to mind the big ignore and continued playing. Her parents were interested in learning a more effective consequence.

The rules of effective commands and command sequence were quickly reviewed. Luis was briefly coached in CDI skills and play commands with Eliana. His skills had improved. He was coached to decrease questions and wait quietly for compliance after giving a command. Eliana was 100% compliant.

Next, the therapist initiated a brief discussion with Eliana's parents about their previous experiences with time-out. Luis noted concerns that time-outs had not been effective for Eliana in the past. Marcos worried about straining his relationship with Eliana and the amount of energy needed to complete time-out. The therapist validated these concerns and introduced the idea of a *therapeutic time-out*. Differences from a typical time-out were discussed. Marcos and Luis expressed understanding that, because of Eliana's special behavioral needs, she would likely benefit from a more structured, predictable time-out. Marcos agreed that continuing daily CDI may help keep their relationship positive while introducing the new discipline procedures. **[Addressing parent's concerns with time-out]**

The therapist taught the family the parent–child interaction therapy time-out procedure for this case. (Please refer to Chapter 8 of this book, the diagrams in Appendix 3 and the PCIT protocol for specifics; Eyberg & Funderburk, 2011.) Eliana's parents planned to use a chair pulled away from the kitchen table, so Eliana could not reach any walls or other objects nearby during time-out at home. Marcos identified Eliana's bedroom as an appropriate back-up space at their home. He planned to remove toys and extra decorations from the room for the next few weeks. Marcos understood that toys in the room could provide extra stimulation, which would work against our goal of having time-out be as boring as possible. Her fathers also appreciated that this would prevent broken toys as had occurred with previous time-outs. Eliana's parents expressed confidence in carrying her to the chair and back-up space if needed. Eliana's grandmother stated that she could not lift Eliana. She was assured that a restriction of privilege could be used in place of the back-up space. The family identified "No more treats at Abue's house today" as an appropriate restriction of privilege. **[Planning time-out and back-up in the home]**

With the therapist coaching through a bug-in-the-ear from behind a two-way mirror, Marcos was coached to explain the time-out procedure to Eliana while showing her the clinic's time-out chair and back-up space. The back-up space was an empty therapy room. It had a small window in the door, so Eliana could see out, and two-way mirror for the therapist and other caregivers to observe. The therapist coached Marcos to gauge Eliana's attention and understanding. Eliana responded correctly to questions about how to avoid time-out ("Listen."), how long time-out on the chair lasted ("3 minutes"), what happened if she got off of the chair early or scooted, tipped, rocked, or stood on the chair ("Go to the room."), how long she had to stay in the room ("1 minute"), and what to do to get out of the room and off of the chair ("Be quiet".). Marcos expressed confidence during this coaching. **[Checking the child's understanding of time-out]**

Marcos was then coached through alternating a couple of minutes of CDI with a simple command with Eliana. During command sequences, Marcos became nervous. He fumbled over his words and apologized to the therapist many times. He also repeatedly asked for clarification on procedures and reassurance about whether he was doing things correctly. Eliana complied with the first command but ignored the second: "Please, put on your mask." (These sessions occurred during the COVID-19 pandemic, and Eliana frequently ignored her father's wishes and took off her face mask when in public). Marcos was coached to wait 5 seconds and say, "If you don't put on your mask, you'll have to sit on the time-out chair." To this, Eliana told her father "No!" Marcos was coached to pick Eliana up quickly from behind and say, "You didn't do what I told you, so you have to sit on the time-out chair." Eliana screamed, tried to run from her father, and kicked her legs when picked up. Marcos was coached to set Eliana's bottom gently on the chair and say, "Stay on the chair until I say you can get off." Before he could finish the statement, Eliana got off the chair and ran across the room laughing. Marcos looked worriedly at the therapist while he was coached to pick up Eliana from behind while giving the *once in a lifetime warning*, "You got off the chair before I said you could. If you get off the chair again, you will go to the time-out room." As soon as Marcos placed Eliana back on the chair, she hopped off of the chair again.

Carrying the child to the back-up space

Marcos was coached to state, "You got off the chair before I said you could, so you have to go to the time-out room." Simultaneously, he was coached to carry Eliana calmly into the back-up room and set her bottom down gently on the floor as far away from the door to the room as possible. He was coached to go out of the room quickly and close the door without pinching Eliana's fingers. Eliana began screaming, crying, and trying to open the door. Marcos was coached to hold the door shut while standing so that Eliana could see his face through the window in the door without making eye contact. The therapist, Luis, and Eliana's grandmother watched Eliana through the two-way mirror to monitor her safety. At this point, Marcos was breathing hard and looking overwhelmed. The therapist coached him through taking a few deep breaths and reminded him that he was not alone. The therapist reiterated that the first time-out would likely be the most demanding and that Eliana would quickly learn to stay in the chair with consistent practice.

Returning the child to the time-out chair

After 1 minute, Eliana was still screaming and crying. Marcos was coached to listen for 5 seconds of silence. After about 5 total minutes in the room, Eliana was quiet for a few seconds. Marcos was coached to enter the room quickly, pick Eliana up gently from behind without speaking, and carry her to the time-out chair. Eliana continued to scream and kick. Marcos was coached to set Eliana's bottom gently down on the chair, step quickly out of Eliana's reach, and say, "Stay on the chair until I say you can get off." Marcos was coached to engage in toy play nearby. Marcos did a great job of describing his play with enthusiasm. The therapist praised him for drawing attention to the contrast between the fun and excitement of toy play with Papi and the boring environment of the time-out chair.

Eliana remained on the chair and began to cry less. However, she was observed sliding her feet out from under herself, gradually shifting her weight off the chair, and watching her father closely for a reaction. After about 1 minute on the chair, the therapist judged that more than half of Eliana's bodyweight was off the chair. Marcos was coached to go to Eliana quickly and quietly, pick her up gently from behind, and carry her to the back-up room. At this, Eliana resumed screaming and crying. Marcos was again coached to set Eliana's bottom down gently on the floor, go quickly out of the room, and hold the door shut while standing so that Eliana could see him.

Again, Marcos breathed hard and wore a worried expression. Eliana continued to cry and scream. She began to scream hurtful statements at her father through the door, for example, "I hate you," "I'm never gonna love you anymore," and "I need a new dad!" This brought tears to Marcos's eyes. The therapist explained through the bug-in-the-ear that it is very common for children to say anything they can think of to get a reaction while in time-out. Eliana continued to make hurtful comments. Now tearful, Marcos told the therapist that he was not sure he could go through with this. The therapist reassured Marcos that he was doing the best thing for his child by not giving in to negative behavior and ultimately teaching her a better way to manage her emotions. She also reminded Marcos that after their first session using time-out, many children return the following week excited to show how well they can listen. **[Disruptive behavior while in the back-up space]** **[Reassuring the caregiver during time-out]**

After about 8 minutes, Eliana quieted for a few seconds. Marcos was coached to enter the room and calmly carry Eliana back to the chair without speaking. The therapist coached Marcos to step quickly away after placing Eliana on the chair saying, "Stay on the chair until I say you can get off." Eliana tried to hit her father, but she could not reach him, and she remained seated on the chair. Again, Marcos was coached to play enthusiastically in hopes of motivating Eliana's desire to return to play.

Eliana's crying gradually ceased, and she sat on the chair for 3 minutes. Marcos was coached to bring Eliana's mask with him while approaching the chair but staying out of Eliana's reach. He was coached to say, "You are sitting quietly on the chair. Are you ready to put on your mask?" Eliana frowned at her father saying, "No!" Marcos was coached to say, "Stay on the chair until I say you can get off," and return to the toys. Eliana responded by screaming and flailing her arms and legs. She remained on the chair for about 30 seconds before trying to leave the room. The therapist quickly blocked the door while coaching Marcos to take Eliana to the back-up space quickly and calmly. **[Returning to the original command]**

Once in the back-up room, Eliana was observed standing in the corner crying. After 1 minute, Eliana continued to cry quietly to herself in the corner. Marcos was coached to return Eliana to the chair as he had done before saying, "Stay on the chair until I say you can get off." This time, Eliana remained on the chair with a sullen look on her face for the full 3 minutes.

Eliana's father was coached to approach her while staying out of reach saying, "You are sitting quietly on the chair. Are you ready to put on your mask?" Eliana grunted while yanking the mask out of her father's hand and putting it on her own face. Marcos smiled broadly and started to speak. The therapist quickly reminded Marcos to stick with a neutral comment like, "Thanks." or "OK." Then he was coached to give another direct instruction: "Now, please take a tissue out of this box." Marcos held out the box to Eliana. While frowning, she yanked out a tissue. The therapist coached Marcos by saying, "Big labeled praise…" In an enthusiastic voice, while grinning from ear to ear, Marcos told Eliana, "Thank you so much for listening, Ellie!" He picked Eliana up, hugging her, and spinning her around in the air. She tried to keep frowning but was **[Neutral comment after compliance with original command]** **[Issuing a follow-up command with labeled praise for compliance]** observed smiling slightly. When her father pointed this out to her, Eliana smiled more and began laughing with her father in spite of herself. Since the original instruction was first given, a total of 33 minutes had elapsed.

Returning to child-directed interaction after time-out

Finally, Marcos was coached to return to CDI. At first, Eliana resisted, but after about 30 seconds, she joined in the play. Marcos was coached to use PRIDE skills for the remainder of the session. After a couple of minutes of this, Eliana began smiling, talking, and playing with her father as happily as she had at the start of the session.

Restriction of privilege if caregiver has physical limitations

Eliana's grandmother and the therapist discussed how she could use restriction of access to treats as a back-up to carrying Eliana to the chair. It was recommended to use the warning, "If you don't sit on the time-out chair, there will be no more treats at Abue's house today." For noncompliance to the warning, she could say, "You didn't do what I told you to, so there will be no snacks at Abue's house today." Eliana's grandmother was encouraged to limit attention for subsequent tantrums or requesting treats. This procedure was reviewed with Eliana as well.

Eliana's caregivers were assigned to continue practicing CDI at home plus 2–4 direct commands during other times of day. Commands would require correct follow-through with a time-out for noncompliance if necessary. The therapist provided hand-outs about how to determine "Is This a Good Time for a Direct Command?" and "Alternatives to Direct Commands" (see Appendix 4). These would guide caregivers in situations when a direct instruction may not be a good idea (e.g., when late for work). On their way out of the clinic, referring to today's time-out, Luis commented that he would not have accepted that behavior from Eliana. The therapist agreed that behavior during the first couple of time-outs is usually intense and that, fortunately, children usually do not respond this way for long. Eliana's caregivers were reminded that children typically learn to control their behavior to avoid or complete time-out quickly in clinic in as few as one to two sessions. It was also explained that by the end of treatment, Eliana should require time-outs rarely, as infrequently as once per week.

9.2.5 Treatment Session 5 (Compliance Training & Time-Out Coaching)

Reviewing at-home compliance training practice

Again, 2 weeks had elapsed since the last session. Eliana's family had missed their last appointment due to car trouble. Eliana entered the clinic talking energetically with her Papi and sat close with him on the couch. Her parents explained that her mood had been more consistently positive over the past 2 weeks than it had previously. Both of Eliana's parents and her grandmother attended this session. They returned a log indicating at-home practice for 10 of the past 14 days. In addition to CDI practice, the log noted that Marcos had given 4 commands for each of the 10 days listed. Eliana was compliant with all commands except on the third and sixth day. These commands had been given at the end of the day when she refused to brush her teeth, even when given the warning statement. The first time, Eliana got off the time-out chair instantly and ran around the house. Marcos carried her to her room where she stayed for 1 minute followed by 9 minutes of waiting until she was quiet for 5 seconds. Eliana then completed her 3-minute chair time-out and complied with the teeth brushing command. On the second occasion, Eliana sat on the time-out chair for the full 3 minutes and subsequently brushed her teeth. Both times, Marcos had forgotten to give a follow-up command.

The focus of this session was on coaching Luis in PDI. Eliana's grandmother again declined coaching. The therapist coached Luis through the bug-in-the-ear to describe the rules of time-out to refresh Eliana's memory. Eliana told her father, "I'm not going to time-out today. I'm gonna listen!" Luis was coached to engage Eliana in CDI. After about 5 minutes, he was coached to give a play command every few minutes. Eliana was 100% compliant without requiring any warnings, and her father gave labeled praises for compliance as instructed. While creating "pancakes" out of yellow Play-Doh, Luis was coached to prompt Eliana that he wanted to play with animals next. He was coached to say, "Put the yellow Play-Doh back in the container." Eliana replied, "In one minute, I just have to finish making the rest." Luis was coached to point from the Play-Doh to the container while remaining quiet for 5 seconds. Since Eliana continued to make pancakes, he was coached to warn her: "If you don't put the yellow Play-Doh back in the container, you'll have to sit on the time-out chair." Eliana became agitated, shaping the Play-Doh more quickly, saying, "I'm almost done!" while Luis remained quiet and pointed for 5 seconds. When Eliana had still not started to put the Play-Doh away, Luis was coached to say, "You did not do what I told you to, so you have to sit on the time-out chair."

Child's second time-out in clinic

Eliana screamed and began stuffing her Play-Doh pancakes into the container. Luis was coached to take the Play-Doh out of her hands and quickly but gently carry her to the chair. Eliana screamed and cried promising that she was ready to pick up now. The therapist coached Luis to ignore this, place Eliana gently on the chair, and tell her, "Stay on the chair until I say you can get off." Before he could finish this statement, Eliana ran back to the table to clean up the Play-Doh. Luis looked to the therapist for direction with a questioning look on his face. The therapist coached Luis to pick up Eliana from behind and carry her to the back-up space. The therapist explained in Luis' earpiece that it might seem overly demanding to expect that Eliana listen within 5 seconds but that if we gave in now, she would learn that she only has to listen after she is sent to time-out.

When Eliana was in the time-out room with the door closed and Luis was standing so she could seem him through the window in the door, Luis looked angry. While Eliana screamed, the therapist asked Luis how he was feeling. He explained that he was frustrated because he found Eliana's behavior acceptable and did not feel that time-out was working for her. The therapist empathized with Luis' frustration. She assured him that, even though it did not seem like it, Eliana was demonstrating signs that she was already learning from this procedure. She had been more willing to listen at this session and at home this week than before starting therapy, according to parent reports. The therapist pointed out that having Luis lead Eliana in a time-out with coaching was actually an important part of treatment, which would help her learning tremendously. Luis agreed to stick with it for at least the remainder of the session.

Addressing parent frustration during time-out

After the required 1 minute in the back-up room, Eliana was quiet. Luis was coached to return her to the chair without speaking. Eliana sat silently on the chair for the full 3 minutes. Her father was coached to approach saying, "You are sitting quietly on the chair. Are you ready to put the yellow Play-Doh in the container?" Eliana ran to the table and quickly put all of the yellow Play-Doh in the container, carefully picking up tiny crumbs that had fallen on the floor without even being asked. Luis was coached to give a neutral comment ("OK.") and issue a follow-up command: "Please, put the blue Play-Doh in its container." Eliana immediately scooped all of the blue Play-Doh into its container and closed the lid. Luis was coached to give an enthusiastic labeled praise for listening *quickly* while rubbing Eliana's back.

After a return to CDI for a few minutes, Luis was coached to issue a direct command every few minutes during play. Eliana complied with all remaining commands. Eliana was observed giggling at her father's "silly" play, climbing on his lap, and specifically offering to share many toys with him.

When asked about his assessment of progress at the end of session, Luis admitted that he was pleased with Eliana's compliance. He explained that he understood that this was a process and that "we didn't get here overnight, so it won't be fixed overnight." Luis and Marcos agreed to stick with the current time-out strategy at home for the next week. They would use direct commands throughout the day as needed and continue with 5 minutes of daily CDI. They agreed to avoid giving direct commands too often and when they were not prepared to follow through with time-out.

9.2.6 Treatment Session 6 (Compliance Coaching, House Rule, & Public Behavior Planning)

Marcos, Eliana, and her grandmother returned to clinic for this session. They reported CDI practice for 6 of the previous 7 days. Both Marcos and Luis had given at least one direct command each day for the past week. Only two warnings were needed and no time-outs were required, as Eliana was 100% compliant. Eliana's grandmother stated that she did not follow the exact rules with giving direct instructions at her house, but Eliana's behavior continued to be good there. It seemed there were few demands on Eliana under her grandmother's care. Marcos explained that Luis was still frustrated that Eliana continued to hit Marcos when she got mad. Tantrums overall had decreased to about three to four times per weekend, but she hit her Papi during every tantrum.

The therapist touched on the idea of incompatible commands. These are commands which cannot be completed while simultaneously engaging in an undesirable target behavior. For instance, if Marcos saw that Eliana was getting upset, he could give her a command to keep her hands in her lap. Then Marcos could follow through with a warning and time-out as needed for noncompliance. This tactic would likely have decreased the frequency of Eliana's hitting as she was highly compliant at this point in treatment. However, this approach would have required Eliana's caregivers to constantly be on alert for *preventing* hitting by looking for signs and giving incompatible commands before hitting occurred.

Alternatively, the idea of a house rule was introduced (Eyberg & Funderburk, 2011). Marcos was enthusiastic and believed Luis would see value in it as well. Marcos and the therapist explained the new house rule to Eliana. They told her that the "no hurting rule" would be instituted at home 1 week from today. For the current week, anytime Eliana hurt (e.g., hit, pinched, kicked) anyone, parents would label it for her (e.g., "You hit me. Remember, next week, if you break the no hurting rule, you'll have to sit on the time-out chair."). Next week, the rule would be enforced. Then, when Eliana intentionally hurt someone, her parent would say, "You broke the no hurting rule, so you have to sit in the time-out chair." Eliana would then be sent to time-out with no warnings. Following completion of time-out, a parent would state, "You are sitting quietly on the chair. Remember, we don't hurt." Her parents would then ignore any arguing or immediate discussion. Marcos felt confident with this plan. **Introducing a house rule**

The therapist also brought up the topic of public behavior. Marcos explained that since Eliana's compliance had improved recently, the family had taken her on several outings without incident. She had been to a grocery store and restaurant without tantrums. Marcos brainstormed strategies for implementing time-out in public if needed. Her father decided that if Eliana was noncompliant with a direct command in a store or restaurant, they could find a place on the floor in an empty aisle or a seat at an empty table for time-out. Marcos believed that even if Eliana screamed, it would be nothing compared to the behavior she had demonstrated in public before. If Eliana refused time-out, her father planned to take her to the car as a back-up space. **Planning for time-out in public**

After a brief session of CDI and PDI coaching, home practice for the week was assigned. Marcos planned to continue with daily CDI in addition to using direct commands as needed throughout the day. He also planned to implement the no hurting house rule. Finally, he and Luis would practice compliance training with proper follow-through in public as needed.

9.2.7 Treatment Session 7 (Follow-Up & Future Planning)

One day before Eliana's next scheduled appointment, the therapist received a phone call from Marcos. He relayed that the continued compliance training, implementation of the house rule, and public behavior plan had been going exceptionally well. Eliana had not required time-out for noncompliance at home or in public. She had only hit her Papi once during the first week of labeling the house rule. Marcos explained that it had been increasingly difficult for him to take time off of work to attend therapy appointments. He requested that their next appointment be scheduled out 3 weeks later to see how things were going at that time. The therapist agreed and let Marcos know the plans for a graduation session, should that be appropriate at the next meeting.

Three weeks later, Eliana, her grandmother, Luis, and Marcos attended treatment for the last time. Eliana reported that she had only been in time-out once over the past month. She had required no public time-outs and had completely stopped all hurting (e.g., hitting, kicking, pinching). All caregivers were pleased and proud of her progress. To celebrate Eliana's success, the family played Eliana's favorite board game together and listening to her favorite music. Eliana was presented with a personalized certificate for "learning to listen." Then everyone described reasons they were proud of Eliana.

Treatment outcomes

At this final session, when asked about how many commands Eliana typically complied with the first time she was told, her parents' answer had changed from 0 to 1 out of 10 at the start of treatment to 9 or 10 out of 10 at the end of treatment. They reported that tantrums and aggression were no longer a problem. Eliana's parents expressed confidence in managing her behavior on their own. Several options for adapting the time-out procedure as Eliana grows were discussed. For example, restriction of privilege can be used instead of a back-up space or even in place of the chair in the future. The family was encouraged to continue using special playtime and especially to return to this daily practice if behavior problems increased in the future.

Planning for the future

10

Further Reading

Books

Cavell, T. A., & Quetsch, L. B. (2023). *Working with parents of aggressive children: A practitioner's guide* (2nd ed.). American Psychological Association.
This book presents a process-oriented framework for conducting therapy with families of children with behavior problems to meet their unique needs. This book highlights methods for goal setting, nurturing the therapeutic alliance, respecting diversity, equity, and inclusion principles, and prioritizing caregivers' health.

Kazdin, A. E., & Weisz, J. R. (Eds.). (2003). *Evidence-based psychotherapies for children and adolescents*. The Guilford Press.
This premiere text on evidence-based treatments for social, emotional, and behavioral concerns in youth provides concise summaries of a comprehensive number of programs. The research base, history, appropriate use, and prominent techniques of each treatment are described, often by leaders in the treatments themselves.

McNeil, C. B., & Hembree-Kigin, T. L. (2010). *Parent–child interaction therapy* (2nd ed.). Springer Science + Business Media.
An in-depth guide to PCIT which includes treatment considerations, extensions to special populations, handouts, and more.

McNeil, C. B., Quetsch, L. B., & Anderson, C. M. (Eds.). (2018). *Handbook of parent-child interaction therapy for children on the autism spectrum*. Springer.
This book is useful for practitioners working with individuals with autism spectrum disorder (ASD) and using a behavioral parent training approach. This unique volume first describes ASD and its treatments, then summarizes parent–child interaction therapy (PCIT), and finally integrates the two, presenting readers with case examples, a theoretical framework, and research to support the use of PCIT for ASD.

Treatment Manuals

Barkley, R. A. (2013). *Defiant children: A clinician's manual for assessment and parent training* (3rd ed.). Guilford Press.

Eyberg, S. M., & Funderburk, B. W. (2011). *Parent–child interaction therapy protocol*. PCIT International.

Forgatch, M. (1994). *Parenting through change: A training manual*. Oregon Social Learning Center.

Gibson, K., Motzenbecker, T., Harvey, C., Han, R. C., & McNeil, C. B. (2021). *Parent–child interaction therapy (PCIT) adapted for older children: A research development manual*. Kindle Direct Publishing. https://www.amazon.com/Parent-Child-Interaction-Therapy-Adapted-Children/dp/B09DJ56QHS

McMahon, R. J., & Forehand, R. L. (2003). *Helping the noncompliant child: Family-based treatment for oppositional behavior* (2nd ed.). Guilford Press.

Pelham, W. E., Greiner, A. R., & Gnagy, E. M. (2019). *Children's Summer Treatment Program manual* [Unpublished manuscript]. Florida International University. https://ccf.fiu.edu/professionals/create-stp/index.html

Websites

Family Interaction Training (FIT) program available at https://www.aucd.org/template/page.cfm?id=1023
Free online training in which clinicians will learn to administer the FIT program to families.

PCIT position statement on time-out available at http://www.pcit.org/pcit-blog/pcit-international-position-statement-on-time-out
Describes the official views of PCIT International, Inc., including definitions and research support.

11

References

Abidin, R. R. (1995). *Parenting stress index: Professional manual* (3rd ed.). Psychological Assessment Resources.

Adams, C. D., & Kelley, M. L. (1992). Managing sibling aggression: Overcorrection as an alternative to time-out. *Behavior Therapy, 23*(4), 707–717. https://doi.org/10.1016/S0005-7894(05)80230-8

Akin, B. A., Lang, K., McDonald, T. P., Yan, Y., & Little, T. (2019). Randomized trial of PMTO in foster care: Six-month child well-being outcomes. *Research on Social Work Practice, 29*(2), 206–222. https://doi.org/10.1177%2F1049731516669822

Alevizos, K. J., & Alevizos, P. N. (1975). The effects of verbalizing contingencies in time-out procedures. *Journal of Behavior Therapy and Experimental Psychiatry, 6*(3), 253–255. https://doi.org/10.1016/0005-7916(75)90113-5

American Academy of Pediatrics, Committee on Psychosocial Aspects of Child and Family Health. (1998). Guidance for effective discipline. *Pediatrics, 101*, 723–728. https://doi.org/10.1542/peds.101.4.723

American Academy of Pediatrics, Council on Child Abuse and Neglect, Committee on Psychosocial Aspects of Child and Family Health. (2018). Effective discipline to raise healthy children. *Pediatrics, 142*(6), Article e20183112 https://doi.org/10.1542/peds.2018-3112

American Counseling Association (ACA). (2014). *2014 ACA code of ethics*. https://www.counseling.org/knowledge-center#2014code

American Medical Association (AMA). (2016). *AMA principles of medical ethics*. https://www.ama-assn.org/delivering-care/ama-principles-medical-ethics

American Psychiatric Association (APA). (2013). *Diagnostic and statistical manual of mental disorders – DSM-5*. https://doi.org/10.1176/appi.books.9780890425596

American Psychological Association (APA). (2017). *Ethical principles of psychologists and code of conduct* [2002, amended effective June 1, 2010, and January 1, 2017]. https://www.apa.org/ethics/code/

Anhalt, K., & Borrego, J. (2010). Ethnic minority children and families. In C. B. McNeil & T. L. Hembree-Kigin (Eds.), *Parent–child interaction therapy* (pp. 363–376). Springer.

Arndorfer, R. E., Allen, K. D., & Aliazireh, L. (1999). Behavioral health needs in pediatric medicine and the acceptability of behavioral solutions: Implications for behavioral psychologists. *Behavior Therapy, 30*(1), 137–148. https://doi.org/10.1016/S0005-7894(99)80050-1

Australian Association for Infant Mental Health (AAIMHI). (2016). *Time out: Position paper 3*. https://www.aaimh.org.au/about-us/position-statements-and-guidelines/

Azrin, N. H., Holz, W. C., & Hake, D. (1963). Fixed-ratio punishment. *Journal of Experimental Analysis of Behavior, 6*(2), 141–148. https://doi.org/10.1901/jeab.1963.6-141

Bandura, A., Ross, D., & Ross, S.A. (1961). Transmission of aggression through imitation of aggressive models. *Journal of Abnormal and Social Psychology, 63*(3), 575–82. https://doi.org/10.1037/h0045925

Barkley, R. A. (2013). *Defiant Children: A clinician's manual for assessment and parent training* (3rd ed.). Guilford Press.

Barkley, R. A. (2014). *Attention-deficit hyperactivity disorder: A handbook for diagnosis and treatment* (4th ed.). The Guilford Press.

Batzer, S., Berg, T., Godinet, M. T., & Stotzer, R. L. (2018). Efficacy or chaos? Parent–child interaction therapy in maltreating populations: A review of research. *Trauma, Violence, & Abuse, 19*(1), 3–19. https://doi.org/10.1177/1524838015620819

Baum, C. G., & Forehand, R. (1981). Long term follow-up assessment of parent training by use of multiple outcome measures. *Behavior Therapy, 12*(5), 643–652. https://doi.org/10.1016/S0005-7894(81)80136-0

Baumrind, D. (1967). Child care practices anteceding three patterns of preschool behaviour. *General Psychology Monograph, 75*, 43–88.

Bean, A. W., & Roberts, M. W. (1981). The effect of time-out release contingencies on changes in child noncompliance. *Journal of Abnormal Child Psychology, 9*(1), 95–105. https://doi.org/10.1007/BF00917860

Benjamin, R., Mazzarins, H., & Kupfersmid, J. (1983). The effect of time-out (TO) duration on assaultiveness in psychiatrically hospitalized children. *Aggressive Behavior, 9*(1), 21–27. https://doi.org/10.1002/1098-2337(1983)9:1<21::AID-AB2480090104>3.0.CO;2-H

Bjørseth, A., Wormdol, A. K., & Chen, Y. (2010). PCIT around the word. In C. B. McNeil & T. L. Hembree-Kigin (Eds.), *Parent–child interaction therapy* (pp. 421–427). Springer.

Blampied, N. M., & Kahan, E. (1992). Acceptability of alternative punishments: A community survey. *Behavior Modification, 16*(3), 400–413. https://doi.org/10.1177/01454455920163006

Brantner, J. P., & Doherty, M. A. (1983). A review of timeout: A conceptual and methodological analysis. In S. Axelrod & J. Apsche (Eds.), *The effects of punishment on human behavior* (pp. 87–132). Guilford Press. https://doi.org/10.1016/B978-0-12-068740-4.50010-6

Broidy, L. M., Nagin, D. S., Tremblay, R. E., Bates, J. E., Brame, B., Dodge, K. A., & Vitaro, F. (2003) Developmental trajectories of childhood disruptive behaviors and adolescent delinquency: A six-site, cross-national study. *Developmental Psychology, 39*(2), 222–245. https://doi.org/10.1037/0012-1649.39.2.222

Bugental, D. B., & Grusec, J. E. (2006). Socialization processes. In N. Eisenberg, W. Damon & R.M. Lerner (Eds.), *Handbook of child psychology: Vol. 3, social, emotional, and personality development* (6th ed., pp. 366–428). John Wiley & Sons Inc.

Burchard, J. D., & Barrera, F. (1972). An analysis of timeout and response cost in a programmed environment. *Journal of Applied Behavior Analysis, 5*(3), 271–282. https://doi.org/10.1901/jaba.1972.5-271

Calhoun, K. S., & Matherne, P. (1975). The effects of varying schedules of time-out on aggressive behavior of a retarded girl. *Journal of Behavior Therapy and Experimental Psychiatry, 6*(2), 139–143. https://doi.org/10.1016/0005-7916(75)90039-7

Capous, D. E., Wallace, N. M., McNeil, D. J., & Cargo, T. A. (2016). Parent–child interaction therapy across diverse cultural groups. In K. Alvarez (Ed.), *Parent–child interactions and relationships: perceptions, practices and developmental outcome* (pp. 1–44). Nova Science Publishers.

Centers for Disease Control and Prevention (CDC). (2019). *Essentials for Parenting Toddlers and Preschoolers: Using time-out*. https://www.cdc.gov/parents/essentials/timeout/index.html

Centers for Disease Control and Prevention (CDC). (2022). *Parent training in behavior management for ADHD*. https://www.cdc.gov/ncbddd/adhd/behavior-therapy.html

Chaffin, M., Funderburk, B., Bard, D., Valle, L. A., & Gurwitch, R. (2011). A combined motivation and parent–child interaction therapy package reduces child welfare recidivism in a randomized dismantling field trial. *Journal of Consulting and Clinical Psychology, 79*(1), 84–95. https://doi.org/10.1037/a0021227

Chaffin, M., Silovsky, J. F., Funderburk, B., Valle, L. A., Brestan, E. V., Balachova, T., Jackson, S., Lensgraf, J., & Bonner, B. L. (2004). Parent–child interaction therapy with physically abusive parents: Efficacy for reducing future abuse reports. *Journal of Consulting and Clinical Psychology, 72*(3), 500–510. https://doi.org/10.1037/0022-006X.72.3.500

Chronis, A. M., Fabiano, G. A., Gnagy, E. M., Onyango, A. N., Pelham, W. E., Jr., Lopez-Williams, A., Chacko, A., Wymbs, B. T., Coles, E. K., & Seymour, K. E. (2004). An evaluation of the Summer Treatment Program for children with attention deficit/hyperactivity disorder using a treatment withdrawal design. *Behavior Therapy, 35*(3), 561–585. https://doi.org.wvu.idm.oclc.org/10.1016/S0005-7894(04)80032-7

Chronis-Tuscano, A., Lewis-Morrarty, E., Woods, K. E., O'Brien, K. A., Mazursky-Horowitz, H., & Thomas, S. R. (2016). Parent–child interaction therapy with emotion coaching for preschoolers with attention-deficit/hyperactivity disorder. *Cognitive and Behavioral Practice, 23*(1), 62–78. https://doi.org/10.1016/j.cbpra.2014.11.001

Chronis-Tuscano, A., Rubin, K. H., O'Brien, K. A., Coplan, R. J., Thomas, S. R., Dougherty, L. R., Cheah, C. S. L., Watts, K., Heverly-Fitt, S., Huggins, S. L., Menzer, M., Begle, A. S., & Wimsatt, M. (2015). Preliminary evaluation of a multimodal early intervention program for behaviorally inhibited preschoolers. *Journal of Consulting and Clinical Psychology, 83*(3), 534–540. https://doi.org/10.1037/a0039043

Cohen, J. A., Berliner, L., & Mannarino, A. (2010). Trauma focused CBT for children with co-occurring trauma and behavior problems. *Child Abuse & Neglect, 34*(4), 215–224. https://doi.org/10.1016/j.chiabu.2009.12.003

Cole, P. M., Martin, S. E., & Dennis, T. A. (2004). Emotion regulation as a scientific construct: Methodological challenges and directions for child development research. *Child Development, 75*(2), 317–333. https://doi.org/10.1111/j.1467-8624.2004.00673.x

Comer, J. S., Chow, C., Chan, P., Cooper-Vince, C., & Wilson, L. A. S. (2013). Psychosocial treatment efficacy for disruptive behavior problems in young children: A meta-analytic examination. *Journal of the American Academy of Child and Adolescent Psychiatry, 52*(1), 26–36. https://doi.org/10.1016/j.jaac.2012.10.001

Corralejo, S. M., Jensen, S. A., & Greathouse, A. D. (2018). Time out for sibling aggression: An analysis of effective durations in a natural setting. *Child & Family Behavior Therapy, 40*(3), 187–203. https://doi.org/10.1080/07317107.2018.1487701

Corralejo, S. M., Jensen, S. A., Greathouse, A. D., & Ward, L. E. (2018). Parameters of time-out: Research update and comparison to parenting programs, books, and online recommendations. *Behavior Therapy, 49*(1), 99–112. https://doi.org/10.1016/j.beth.2017.09.005

Dadds, M. R., Adlington, F. M., & Christensen, A. P. (1987). Children's perceptions of time out and other maternal disciplinary strategies: The effects of clinic status and exposure to behavioural treatment. *Behaviour Change, 4*(4), 3–13. https://doi.org/10.1017/S0813483900008275

Dadds, M. R., & Tully, L. A. (2019). What is it to discipline a child: What should it be? A reanalysis of time-out from the perspective of child mental health, attachment, and trauma. *American Psychologist, 74*(7), 794–808. https://doi.org/10.1037/amp0000449

Day, D. E., & Roberts, M. W. (1983). An analysis of the physical punishment component of a parent training program. *Journal of Abnormal Child Psychology, 11*, 141–152. https://doi.org/10.1007/BF00912184

Deci, E. L., & Ryan, R. M. (1985). *Intrinsic motivation and self-determination in human behavior*. Plenum Press. https://doi.org/10.1007/978-1-4899-2271-7

Diamond, A. (2002). Normal development of prefrontal cortex from birth to young adulthood: Cognitive functions, anatomy, and biochemistry. In D. T. Stuss & R. T. Knight (Eds.), *Principles of frontal lobe function* (pp. 466–503). Oxford University Press. https://doi.org/10.1093/acprof:oso/9780195134971.003.0029

Dishion, T., Forgatch, M., Chamberlain, P., & Pelham, W. E. (2016). The Oregon model of behavior family therapy: From intervention design to promoting large-scale system change. *Behavior Therapy, 47*(6), 812–837. https://doi.org/10.1016/j.beth.2016.02.002

Donaldson, J. M., & Vollmer, T. R. (2011). An evaluation and comparison of time-out procedures with and without release contingencies. *Journal of Applied Behavior Analysis, 44*(4), 693–705. https://doi.org/10.1901/jaba.2011.44-693

Donaldson, J. M., Vollmer, T. R., Yakich, T. M., & Van Camp, C. (2013). Effects of a reduced time-out interval on compliance with the time-out instruction. *Journal of Applied Behavior Analysis, 46*(2), 369–378. https://doi.org/10.1002/jaba.40

Drayton, A. K., Andersen, M. N., Knight, R. M., Felt, B. T., Fredericks, E. M., & Dore-Stites, D. J. (2014). Internet guidance on time out. *Journal of Developmental & Behavioral Pediatrics, 35*(4), 239–246. https://doi.org/10.1097/DBP.0000000000000059

Eaves, S. H., Sheperis, C. J., Blanchard, T., Baylot, L., & Doggett, R. A. (2005). Teaching time-out and job card grounding procedures to parents: A primer for family counselors. *The Family Journal, 13*(3), 252–258. https://doi.org/10.1177/1066480704273638

Eisenberger, N. I., Lieberman, M. D., & Williams, K. D. (2003). Does rejection hurt? An FMRI study of social exclusion. *Science, 302*(5643), 290–292. https://doi.org/10.1126/science.1089134

Eisenstadt, T. H., Eyberg, S., McNeil, C. B., Newcomb, K., & Funderburk, B. (1993). Parent–child interaction therapy with behavior problem children: Relative effectiveness of two stages and overall treatment outcome. *Journal of Clinical Child Psychology, 22*(1), 42–51. https://doi.org/10.1207/s15374424jccp2201_4

Erford, B. T. (1999). A modified time-out procedure for children with noncompliant or defiant behaviors. *Professional School Counseling, 2*(3), 205–210.

Everett, G. E., Hupp, S. D. A., & Olmi, D. J. (2010). Time-out with parents: A descriptive analysis of 30 years of research. *Education & Treatment of Children, 33*(2), 235–259. https://doi.org/10.1353/etc.0.0091

Everett, G. E., Olmi, D. J., Edwards, R. P., Tingstrom, D. H., Sterling-Turner, H. E., & Christ, T. J. (2007). An empirical investigation of time-out with and without escape extinction to treat escape-maintained noncompliance. *Behavior Modification, 31*(4), 412–434. https://doi.org/10.1177/0145445506297725

Eyberg, S. M., & Funderburk, B. W. (2011). *Parent–child interaction therapy protocol*. PCIT International.

Eyberg, S. M., Nelson, M. M., & Boggs, S. R. (2008). Evidence-based psychosocial treatments for children and adolescents with disruptive behavior. *Journal of Clinical Child and Adolescent Psychology, 37*(1), 215–237. https://doi.org/10.1080/15374410701820117

Fabiano, G. A., Pelham, W. E., Jr., Manos, M. J., Gnagy, E. M., Chronis, A. M., Onyango, A. N., Lopez-Williams, A., Burrows-MacLean, L., Coles, E. K., Meichenbaum, D. L., Caserta, D. A., & Swain, S. (2004). An evaluation of three time-out procedures for children with attention deficit/hyperactivity disorder. *Behavior Therapy, 35*(3), 449–469. https://doi.org/10.1016/S0005-7894(04)80027-3

Fabiano, G. A., Schatz, N. K., & Pelham, W. E., Jr. (2014). Summer treatment programs for youth with ADHD. *Child and Adolescent Psychiatric Clinics of North America, 23*(4), 757–773. https://doi.org/10.1016/j.chc.2014.05.012

Ferster, C. B. (1958). Control of behavior in chimpanzees and pigeons by time out from positive reinforcement. *Psychological Monographs: General and Applied, 72*(8), 1–38. https://doi.org/10.1037/h0093787

Ferster, C. B., & Skinner, B. F. (1957). *Schedules of reinforcement*. Appleton. https://doi.org/10.1037/10627-000

Flora, S. R. (1990). Undermining intrinsic interest from the standpoint of a behaviorist. *The Psychological Record, 40*(3), 323–346. https://doi.org/10.1007/BF03399544

Fontes, R. M., & Shahan, T. A. (2020). Punishment and its putative fallout: A reappraisal. *Journal of the Experimental Analysis of Behavior, 115*(1), 185–203. https://doi.org/10.1002/jeab.653

Forcino, S. S., Nadler, C. B., & Roberts, M. W. (2019). Parent training for middle childhood conduct problems: Child opposition to timeout and token fines. *Practice Innovations, 4*(1), 1–12. https://doi.org/10.1037/pri0000090

Forehand, R., & Long, N. (2010). *Parenting the strong-willed child: The clinically proven five-week program for parents of two- to six-year-olds* (3rd ed.). McGraw Hill Professional.

Forehand, R., & McKinney, B. (1993). Historical overview of child discipline in the United States: Implications for mental health clinicians and researchers. *Journal of Child and Family Studies, 2*(3), 221–228. https://doi.org/10.1007/BF01321332

Forehand, R., Roberts, M. W., Doleys, D. M., Hobbs, S. A., & Resick, P. A. (1976). An examination of disciplinary procedures with children. *Journal of Experimental Child Psychology, 21*(1), 109–120. https://doi.org/10.1016/0022-0965(76)90061-8

Forgatch, M. S., & Gewirtz, A. H. (2017). The evolution of the Oregon model of parent management training: An intervention for antisocial behavior in children and adolescents. In

J. R. Weisz & A. E. Kazdin (Eds.), *Evidence-based psychotherapies for children and adolescents* (3rd ed., pp. 85–102). The Guilford Press.

Forgatch, M. S., & Patterson, G. R. (2010). Parent Management Training–Oregon model: An intervention for antisocial behavior in children and adolescents. In J. R. Weisz & A. E. Kazdin (Eds.), *Evidence-based psychotherapies for children and adolescents* (2nd ed., pp. 159–177). The Guilford Press.

Foxx, R. M., & Shapiro, S. T. (1978). The timeout ribbon: A nonexclusionary timeout procedure. *Journal of Applied Behavior Analysis, 11*(1), 125–136. https://doi.org/10.1901/jaba.1978.11-125

Freeman, B. J., Somerset, T., & Ritvo, E. R. (1976). Effect of duration of time out in suppressing disruptive behavior of a severely autistic child. *Psychological Reports, 38*(1), 124–126. https://doi.org/10.2466/pr0.1976.38.1.124

Gardner, H., Forehand, R., & Roberts, M. W. (1976). Timeout with children: Effects of an explanation and brief parent training on child and parent behaviors. *Journal of Abnormal Child Psychology, 4*, 277–288. https://doi.org/10.1007/BF00917764

Gartrell, D. (1994). *A guidance approach to discipline*. Delmar.

Gartrell, D. (2001). Replacing time-out: Part one – Using guidance to build an encouraging classroom. *Young Children, 56*(6), 8–16.

Gartrell, D. (2002). Replacing time-out; Part two – Using guidance to maintain an encouraging classroom. *Young Children, 57*(2), 36–39.

Gershoff, E. T. (2002). Corporal punishment by parents and associated child behaviors and experiences: A meta-analytic and theoretical review. *Psychological Bulletin, 128*(4), 539–579. https://doi.org/10.1037/0033-2909.128.4.539

Gershoff, E. T., & Bitensky, S. H. (2007). The case against corporal punishment of children: Converging evidence from social science research and international human rights law and implications for US public policy. *Psychology, Public Policy, and Law, 13*(4), 231–272. https://doi.org/10.1037/1076-8971.13.4.231

Gershoff, E. T., Grogan-Kaylor, A., Lansford, J. E., Chang, L., Zelli, A., Deater-Deckard, K., & Dodge, K. A. (2010). Parent discipline practices in an international sample: Associations with child behaviors and moderation by perceived normativeness. *Child Development, 81*(2), 487–502. https://doi.org/10.1111/j.1467-8624.2009.01409.x

Gibson, K., Motzenbecker, T., Harvey, C., Han, R. C., & McNeil, C. B. (2022). *Parent–child interaction therapy (PCIT) adapted for older children: A research development manual*. Kindle Direct Publishing.

Gilliom, M., Shaw, D. S., Beck, J. E., Schonberg, M. A., & Lukon, J. L. (2002). Anger regulation in disadvantaged preschool boys: Strategies, antecedents, and the development of self-control. *Developmental Psychology, 38*(2), 222–235. https://doi.org/10.1037/0012-1649.38.2.222.

Girard, E. I., Wallace, N. M., Kohlhoff, J. R., Morgan, S. S. J., & McNeil, C. B. (2018). *Parent–child interaction therapy with toddlers: Improving attachment and emotion regulation*. Springer. https://doi.org/10.1007/978-3-319-93251-4

Global Initiative to End All Corporal Punishment of Children. (2020a). *Corporal punishment of children in the United States*. http://www.endcorporalpunishment.org/wp-content/uploads/country-reports/USA.pdf

Global Initiative to End All Corporal Punishment of Children. (2020b). *Global report 2019: Progress towards ending corporal punishment of children*. https://endcorporalpunishment.org/resources/global-report-2019/

Gordon, T. (2000). *Parent Effectiveness Training: The proven program for raising responsible children*. Three Rivers Press.

Greene, R. J., Hoats, D. L., & Hornick, A. J. (1970). Music distortion: A new technique for behavior modification. *The Psychological Record, 20*, 107–109. https://doi.org/10.1007/BF03393917

Greene, R. W. (1998). *The explosive child: A new approach for understanding and parenting easily frustrated, "chronically inflexible" children*. HarperCollins.

Grusec, J. E., Danyliuk, T., Kil, H., & O'Neill, D. (2017). Perspectives on parent discipline and child outcomes. *International Journal of Behavioral Development, 41*(4), 465–471. https://doi.org/10.1177/0165025416681538

Hanf, C. (1969). *A two-stage program for modifying maternal controlling during mother–child (M–C) interaction*. Paper presented at the meeting of the Western Psychological Association, Vancouver, BC, Canada.

Harris, K. R. (1985). Definitional, parametric, and procedural considerations in timeout interventions and research. *Exceptional Children, 51*(4), 279–288. https://doi.org/10.1177/001440298405100403

Harris, S. L., & Ersner-Hershfield, R. (1978). Behavioral suppression of seriously disruptive behavior in psychotic and retarded patients: A review of punishment and its alternatives. *Psychological Bulletin, 85*(6), 1352–1375. https://doi.org/10.1037/0033-2909.85.6.1352

Havighurst, S. S., Wilson, K. R., Harley, A. E., Kehoe, C., Efron, D., & Prior, M. R. (2013). "Tuning into Kids": Reducing young children's behavior problems using an emotion coaching parenting program. *Child Psychiatry & Human Development, 44*, 247–264. https://doi.org/10.1007/s10578-012-0322-1

Hernstein, R. J. (1955). *Behavioral consequences of the removal of a discriminative stimulus associated with variable-interval reinforcement* [Unpublished doctoral dissertation]. Harvard University.

Hobbs, S. A., & Forehand, R. (1975). Effects of differential release from time-out on children's deviant behavior. *Journal of Behavior Therapy and Experimental Psychiatry, 6*(3), 256-257. https://doi.org/10.1016/0005-7916(75)90114-7

Hobbs, S. A., & Forehand, R. (1977). Important parameters in the use of timeout with children: A re-examination. *Journal of Behavior Therapy and Experimental Psychiatry, 8*(4), 365–370. https://doi.org/10.1016/0005-7916(77)90004-0

Hobbs, S. A., Forehand, R., & Murray, R. G. (1978). Effects of various durations of time-out on the noncompliant behavior of children. *Behavior Therapy, 9*(4), 652–656. https://doi.org/10.1016/S0005-7894(78)80142-7

Hobbs, S. A., Walle, D. L., & Caldwell, H. S. (1984). Maternal evaluation of social reinforcement and time-out: Effects of brief parent training. *Journal of Consulting and Clinical Psychology, 52*(1), 135–136. https://doi.org/10.1037/0022-006X.52.1.135f

Hood, K. K., & Eyberg, S. M. (2003). Outcomes of parent–child interaction therapy: Mothers' reports of maintenance three to six years after treatment. *Journal of Clinical Child and Adolescent Psychology, 32*(3), 419–429. https://doi.org/10.1207/S15374424JCCP3203_10

James, J. E. (1976). The influence of duration on the effects of time-out from speaking. *Journal of Speech, Language, and Hearing Research, 19*(2), 206–215. https://doi.org/10.1044/jshr.1902.206

Joint Commission on Accreditation of Healthcare Organizations. (2009). *Joint Commission standards on restraint and seclusion/nonviolent intervention training program*. Joint-Commission-Restraint-Seclusion-Alignment-2011.pdf (crisisprevention.com)

Jones, M. L., Eyberg, S. M., Adams, C. D., & Boggs, S. R. (1998). Treatment acceptability of behavioral interventions for children: An assessment by mothers of children with disruptive behavior disorders. *Child & Family Behavior Therapy, 20*(4), 15–26. https://doi.org/10.1300/J019v20n04_02

Jones, R. N., Sloane, H. N., & Roberts, M. W. (1992). Limitations of "don't" instructional control. *Behavior Therapy, 23*(1), 131–140. https://doi.org/10.1016/s0005-7894(05)80313-2

Kaminski, J., & Claussen, A. (2017). Evidence based update for psychosocial treatments for disruptive behaviors in children. *Journal of Clinical Child and Adolescent Psychology, 46*(4), 477–499. https://doi.org/10.1080/15374416.2017.1310044

Kaminski, J. W., Valle, L. A., Filene, J. H., & Boyle, C. L. (2008). A meta-analytic review of components associated with parent training program effectiveness. *Journal of Abnormal Child Psychology, 36*(4), 567–89. https://doi.org/10.1007/s10802-007-9201-9

Kapalka, G. M., & Bryk, L. J. (2007). Two- to four-minute time-out is sufficient for young boys with ADHD. *Early Childhood Services: An Interdisciplinary Journal of Effectiveness, 1*(3), 181–188.

Katz, B. R., & Lattal, K. A. (2021). What is an extinction burst? A case study in the analysis of transitional behavior. *Journal of the Experimental Analysis of Behavior, 115*(1), 129–140. https://doi.org/10.1002/jeab.642

Kauffman Best Practices Project to Help Children Heal From Child Abuse. (2004). *Kauffman Best Practices Project Final Report: Closing the quality chasm in child abuse treatment; identifying and disseminating best practices*. https://depts.washington.edu/uwhatc/PDF/kauffmanfinal.pdf

Kazdin, A. E. (1980). Acceptability of time out from reinforcement procedures for disruptive child behavior. *Behavior Therapy, 11*(3), 329–344. https://doi.org/10.1016/S0005-7894(80)80050-5

Kazdin, A. E. (2005). *Parent management training: Treatment for oppositional, aggressive, and antisocial behavior in children and adolescents* (3rd ed.). Oxford University Press.

Kazdin, A. E. (2008). *The Kazdin method for parenting the defiant child: With no pills, no therapy, no contest of wills*. Houghton Mifflin Company.

Kazdin, A. E. (2017). Parent management training and problem-solving skills training for child and adolescent conduct problems. In J. R. Weisz & A. E. Kazdin (Eds.), *Evidence-based psychotherapies for children and adolescents* (3rd ed., pp. 142–158). The Guilford Press.

Kazdin, A. E., & Benjet, C. (2003). Spanking children: Evidence and issues. *Current Directions in Psychological Science, 12*(3), 99–103. https://doi.org/10.1111/1467-8721.01239

Kelley, M. L., Power, T. G., & Wimbush, D. D. (1992). Determinants of disciplinary practices in low-income Black mothers. *Child Development, 63*(3), 573–582. https://doi.org/10.2307/1131347

Kendall, P. C., Nay, W. R., & Jeffers, J. (1975). Timeout duration and contrast effects: A systematic evaluation of a successive treatments design. *Behavior Therapy, 6*(5), 609–615. https://doi.org/10.1016/S0005-7894(75)80182-1

Kim, E., & Hong, S. (2007). First generation Korean American parents' perceptions of discipline. *Journal of Professional Nursing, 23* (1), 60-68. https://doi.org/10.1016/j.profnurs.2006.12.002

Knight, R. M., Albright, J., Deling, L., Dore-Stites, D., & Drayton, A. K. (2020). Longitudinal relationship between time-out and child emotional and behavioral functioning. *Journal of Developmental and Behavioral Pediatrics, 41*(1), 31–37. https://doi.org/10.1097/DBP.0000000000000725

Kohn, A. (1993). *Punished by rewards: The trouble with gold stars, incentive plans, a's, praise, and other bribes*. Houghton Mifflin.

Kolko, D. J., Herschell, A. D., Baumann, B. L., Hart, J. A., & Wisniewski, S. R. (2018). AF-CBT for families experiencing physical aggression or abuse served by the mental health or child welfare system: An effectiveness trial. *Child Maltreatment, 23*(4), 319–333. https://doi.org/10.1177/1077559518781068

Kunkle, K. L., & Ortiz, C. (2016). Maternal treatment acceptability and preference of room time-out and deferred time-out escape contingencies. *Child & Family Behavior Therapy, 38*(2), 105–123. https://doi.org/10.1080/07317107.2016.1172875

Larson, K. L., Ayllon, T., & Barrett, D. H. (1987). A behavioral feeding program for failure-to-thrive infants. *Behaviour Research and Therapy, 25*(1), 39–47. https://doi.org/10.1016/0005-7967(87)90113-6

Larzelere, R. E., Gunnoe, M. L., Roberts, M. W., Lin, H., & Ferguson, C. J. (2020). Causal evidence for exclusively positive parenting and for timeout: Rejoinder to Holden, Grogan-Kaylor, Durrant, and Gershoff (2017). *Marriage & Family Review, 56*(4), 287–319. https://doi.org/10.1080/01494929.2020.1712304

Lavigueur, H., Peterson, R. F., Sheese, J. G., & Peterson, L. W. (1973). Behavioral treatment in the home: Effects on an untreated sibling and long-term follow-up. *Behavior Therapy, 4*(3), 431–441. https://doi.org/10.1016/S0005-7894(73)80125-X

Lenze, S. N., Pautsch, J., & Luby, J. (2011). Parent–child interaction therapy emotion development: A novel treatment for depression in preschool children. *Depression and Anxiety, 28*(2), 153–159. https://doi.org/10.1002/da.20770

Lieneman, C., Girard, E., Quetsch, L., & McNeil, C. (2020). Emotion regulation and attrition in parent–child interaction therapy. *Journal of Child and Family Studies, 29*, 978-996. https://doi.org/10.1007/s10826-019-01674-4

Lieneman, C., Ruckle, M., & McNeil, C. (2019). Parent–child interaction therapy for a child with autism spectrum disorder: A case study examining effects on ASD symptoms, social engagement, pretend play, and disruptive behavior. In C. B. McNeil, L. B. Quetsch, & C. M. Anderson (Eds.), *Handbook of parent–child interaction therapy for children on the autism spectrum* (pp. 677-696). Springer.

Long, P., Forehand, R., Wierson, M., & Morgan, A. (1994). Does parent training with young noncompliant children have long-term effects? *Behaviour Research and Therapy, 32*(1), 101–107. https://doi.org/10.1016/0005-7967(94)90088-4

Luiselli, J. K., Pace, G. M., & Dunn, E. K. (2006). Effects of behavior-contingent and fixed-time release contingencies on frequency and duration of therapeutic restraint. *Behavior Modification, 30*(4), 442–455. https://doi.org/10.1177/0145445504267400

Lundahl, B., Risser, H. J., & Lovejoy, M. C. (2006). A meta-analysis of parent training: Moderators and follow-up effects. *Clinical Psychology Review, 26*(1), 86–104. https://doi.org/10.1016/j.cpr.2005.07.004

MacDonough, T. S., & Forehand, R. (1973). Response-contingent time out: Important parameters in behavior modification with children. *Journal of Behavior Therapy and Experimental Psychiatry, 4*(3), 231–236. https://doi.org/10.1016/0005-7916(73)90079-7

Mace, F. C., & Heller, M. (1990). A comparison of exclusion time-out and contingent observation for reducing severe disruptive behavior in a 7 year old boy. *Child & Family Behavior Therapy, 12*(1), 57–68. https://doi.org/10.1300/J019v12n01_04

Mace, F. C., Page, T. J., Ivancic, M. T., & O'Brien, S. (1986). Effectiveness of brief time-out with and without contingent delay: A comparative analysis. *Journal of Applied Behavior Analysis, 19*(1), 79–86. https://doi.org/10.1901/jaba.1986.19-79

Magee, S. K., & Ellis, J. (2001). The detrimental effects of physical restraint as a consequence for inappropriate classroom behavior. *Journal of Applied Behavior Analysis, 34*(4), 501–504. https://doi.org/10.1901/jaba.2001.34-501

Martin, R. R., & Hasbrouck, J. M. (1977). The effects of punishment schedule on disfluency rate. *Language and Speech, 20*(2), 127–135. https://doi.org/10.1177/002383097702000204

Masse, J., & Girard, E. (n.d.). *PCIT time-out flip book*. PCIT International.

Mathews, J. R., Friman, P. C., Barone, V. J., Ross, L. V., & Christophersen, E. R. (1987). Decreasing dangerous infant behaviors through parent instruction. *Journal of Applied Behavior Analysis, 20*(2), 165–169. https://doi.org/10.1901/jaba.1987.20-165

Matos, M., Torres, R., Santiago, R., Jurado, M., & Rodrigues, I. (2006). Adaptation of parent–child interaction therapy for Puerto Rican families: A preliminary study. *Family Process, 45*, 203-222. https://doi.org/10.1111/j.1545-5300.2006.00091.x

Matsumoto, Y., Sofronoff, K., & Sanders, M. R. (2007). The efficacy and acceptability of the Triple P – Positive Parenting Program with Japanese parents. *Behaviour Change, 24*(4), 205–218. https://doi.org/10.1375/bech.24.4.205

Mazurek, M. O., Kanne, S. M., & Wodka, E. L. (2013). Physical aggression in children and adolescents with autism spectrum disorders. *Research in Autism Spectrum Disorders, 7*(3), 455–465. https://doi.org/10.1016/j.rasd.2012.11.004

McCabe, K. M., Yeh, M., & Zerr, A. A. (2020). Personalizing behavioral parent training Interventions to Improve treatment engagement and outcomes for culturally diverse families. *Psychology Research and Behavior Management, 13*, 41–53. https://doi.org/10.2147/PRBM.S230005

McEvoy, M., Lee, C., O'Neill, A., Groisman, A., Roberts-Butelman, K., Dinghra, K., & Porder, K. (2005). Are there universal parenting concepts among culturally diverse families in an inner-city pediatric clinic? *Journal of Pediatric Health Care: Official Publication of National Association of Pediatric Nurse Associates & Practitioners, 19*(3), 142–150. https://doi.org/10.1016/j.pedhc.2004.10.007

McGuffin, P. W. (1991). The effect of timeout duration on frequency of aggression in hospitalized children with conduct disorders. *Behavioral Residential Treatment, 6*(4), 279–288. https://doi.org/10.1002/bin.2360060405

McMahon, R. J., & Forehand, R. L. (2003). *Helping the noncompliant child: Family-based treatment for oppositional behavior* (2nd ed.). Guilford Press.

McMillan, D. E. (1967). A comparison of the punishing effects of response-produced shock and response produced time out. *Journal of the Experimental Analysis of Behavior, 10*(5), 439– 449. https://doi.org/10.1901/jeab.1967.10-439

McNeil, C. B., Clemens-Mowrer, L., Gurwitch, R. H., & Funderburk, B. W. (1994). Assessment of a new procedure to prevent timeout escape in preschoolers. *Child & Family Behavior Therapy, 16*(3), 27–35. https://doi.org/10.1300/J019v16n03_04

McNeil, C. B., & Hembree-Kigin, T. L. (2010). *Parent–child interaction therapy* (2nd ed.). Springer Science + Business Media. https://doi.org/10.1007/978-0-387-88639-8

McNeil, C. B., Quetsch, L. B., & Anderson, C. M. (Eds.). (2018). *Handbook of parent–child interaction therapy for children on the autism spectrum*. Springer. https://doi.org/10.1007/978-3-030-03213-5

Miles, C. L., & Cuvo, A. J. (1980). Modification of the disruptive and productive classroom behavior of a severely retarded child: A comparison of two procedures. *Education and Treatment of Children, 3*, 113–121.

Ministry of Health NZ. (2019). *Interim position statement – Use of time-out in ICAMHS settings*. https://wharaurau.org.nz/resources/news/moh-interim-position-statement-use-time-out-icamhs-settings-20190315

Morawska, A., & Sanders, M. (2011). Parental use of time out revisited: A useful or harmful parenting strategy? *Journal of Child and Family Studies, 20*(1), 1–8. https://doi.org/10.1007/s10826-010-9371-x

Nelson, D. M., & Rutherford, R. B. (1983). Timeout revisited: Guidelines for its use in special education. *Exceptional Education Quarterly, 3*(4), 56–67. https://doi.org/10.1177/074193258300300412

Nixon, R. D. V., Sweeney, L., Erickson, D. B., & Touyz, S. W. (2003). Parent–child interaction therapy: A comparison of standard and abbreviated treatments for oppositional defiant children. *Journal of Consulting and Clinical Psychology, 71*(2), 251–260. https://doi.org/10.1037/0022-006x.71.2.251

Novotney, A. (2012). Parenting that works: Seven research-backed ways to improve parenting. *Monitor on Psychology, 43*(9). http://www.apa.org/monitor/2012/10/parenting.aspx

Ollendick, T. H., Greene, R. W., Austin, K. E., Fraire, M. G., Halldorsdottir, T., Allen, K. B., Jarrett, M. A., Lewis, K. M., Whitmore Smith, M., Cunningham, N. R., Noguchi, R. J. P., Canavera, K., & Wolff, J. C. (2016). Parent management training and collaborative & proactive solutions: A randomized control trial for oppositional youth. *Journal of Clinical Child and Adolescent Psychology, 45*(5), 591–604. https://doi.org/10.1080/15374416.2015.1004681

Passini, C. M., Pihet, S., & Favez, N. (2014). Assessing specific discipline techniques: A mixed-methods approach. *Journal of Child and Family Studies, 23*(8), 1389–1402. https://doi.org/10.1007/s10826-013-9796-0

Patterson, G. R. (1979). A performance theory for coercive family interaction. In R. B. Cairns (Ed.), *The analysis of social interactions: Methods, issues, and illustrations* (pp. 119–162). Lawrence Erlbaum.

Patterson, G. R. (2005). The next generation of PMTO models. *The Behavior Therapist, 28*(2), 27–33.

Patterson, G. R., & White, G. D. (1969). It's a small world: The application of "timeout from positive reinforcement." *Oregon Psychological Association Newsletter, 15*(2).

Pearl, E., Thieken, L., Olafson, E., Boat, B., Connelly, L., Barnes, J., & Putnam, F. (2012). Effectiveness of community dissemination of parent–child interaction therapy. *Psychological Trauma: Theory, Research, Practice, and Policy, 4*(2), 204–213. https://doi.org/10.1037/a0022948

Pelham, W. E., Greiner, A. R., & Gnagy, E. M. (2019). *Children's Summer Treatment Program manual* [Unpublished manuscript]. Center for Children and Families, Florida International University.

Pelham, W. E., Wheeler, T., & Chronis, A. (1998). Empirically supported psychosocial treatments for attention deficit hyperactivity disorder. *Journal of Clinical Child Psychology, 27*(2), 190-205. https://doi.org/10.1207/s15374424jccp2702_6

Pendergrass, V. E. (1971). Effects of length of time-out from positive reinforcement and schedule of application in suppression of aggressive behavior. *Psychological Record, 21,* 75–80. https://doi.org/10.1007/BF03393992

Pincus, D. B., Santucci, L. C., Ehrenreich, J. T., & Eyberg, S. M. (2008). The implementation of modified parent–child interaction therapy for youth with separation anxiety disorder. *Cognitive and Behavioral Practice, 15*(2), 118–125. https://doi.org/10.1016/j.cbpra.2007.08.002

Porterfield, J. K., Herbert-Jackson, E., & Risley, T. R. (1976). Contingent observation: An effective and acceptable procedure for reducing disruptive behavior of young children in a group setting. *Journal of Applied Behavior Analysis, 9*(1), 55–64. https://doi.org/10.1901/jaba.1976.9-55

Puliafico, A. C., Comer, J. S., & Pincus, D. B. (2012). Adapting parent–child interaction therapy to treat anxiety disorders in young children. *Child and Adolescent Psychiatric Clinics of North America, 21*(3), 607–619. https://doi.org/10.1016/j.chc.2012.05.005

Quetsch, L. B., Lieneman, C., & McNeil, C. (2017). *The role of time-out in trauma-informed treatment for young children.* https://societyforpsychotherapy.org/role-time-trauma-informed-treatment-young-children/

Quetsch, L. B., Wallace, N. M., Herschell, A. D., & McNeil, C. B. (2015). Weighing in on the time-out controversy: An empirical perspective. *The Clinical Psychologist, 68*(2), 4–19.

Regalado, M., Sareen, H., Inkelas, M., Wissow, L. S., & Halfon, N. (2004). Parents' discipline of young children: Results from the National Survey of Early Childhood Health. *Pediatrics, 133*(6 Suppl), 1952–1958. https://doi.org/10.1542/peds.113.S5.1952

Reid, J. B., Patterson, G. R., & Snyder, J. (2002). *Antisocial behavior in children and adolescents: A developmental analysis and model for intervention.* American Psychological Association. https://doi.org/10.1037/10468-000

Reitman, D. (1998). Punished by misunderstanding: A critical evaluation of Kohn's punished by rewards and its implications for behavioral interventions with children. *The Behavior Analyst, 21,* 143–157. https://doi.org/10.1007/BF03392789

Reitman, D., & McMahon, R. J. (2013). Constance "Connie" Hanf (1917–2002): The mentor and the model. *Cognitive and Behavioral Practice, 20*(1), 106–116. https://doi.org/10.1016/j.cbpra.2012.02.005

Risley, T. R. (1968). The effects and side effects of punishing the autistic behaviors of a deviant child. *Journal of Applied Behavior, 1*(1), 21–34. https://doi.org/10.1901/jaba.1968.1-21

Roberts, M. W. (1982). The effects of warned versus unwarned time-out procedures on child noncompliance. *Child & Family Behavior Therapy, 4*(1), 37–53. https://doi.org/10.1300/J019v04n01_04

Roberts, M. W. (1988). Enforcing chair timeouts with room timeouts. *Behavior Modification, 12*(3), 353–370. https://doi.org/10.1177/01454455880123003

Roberts, M. W., & Powers, S. W. (1990). Adjusting chair timeout enforcement procedures for oppositional children. *Behavior Therapy, 21*(3), 257–271. https://doi.org/10.1016/S0005-7894(05)80329-6

Rodgers, A. Y. (1992). Acceptability of time out procedures for school age children: Evaluations by direct care staff and students in child development and child care. *Child and Youth Care Forum, 21,* 195–208. https://doi.org/10.1007/BF00757570

Rolider, A., & Van Houten, R. (1985). Movement suppression time-out for undesirable behavior in psychotic and severely developmentally delayed children. *Journal of Applied Behavior Analysis, 18*(4), 275–288. https://doi.org/10.1901/jaba.1985.18-275

Ryan, R. M., Kalil, A., Ziol-Guest, K. M., & Padilla, C. (2016). Socioeconomic gaps in parents' discipline strategies from 1988 to 2011. *Pediatrics, 138*(6), Article e20160720. https://doi.org/10.1542/peds.2016-0720

Sanders, M. R. (1999). Triple P – Positive Parenting Program: Towards an empirically validated multilevel parenting and family support strategy for the prevention of behavior and emotional problems in children. *Clinical Child and Family Psychology Review, 2*(2), 91–90. https://doi.org/10.1023/a:1021843613840

Sanders, M. R. (2008). Triple P – Positive Parenting Program as a public health approach to strengthening parenting. *Journal of Family Psychology, 22*(4), 506–517. https://doi.org/10.1037/0893-3200.22.3.506

Sanders, M. R., Markie-Dadds, C., & Turner, K. M. T. (2003). Theoretical, scientific and clinical foundations of the Triple P-Positive Parenting Program: A population approach to the promotion of parenting competence. *Parenting Research and Practice Monograph, 1*, 1–21. https://doi.org/10.1002/car.798

Sanders, M. R., Montgomery, D. T., & Brechman-Toussaint, M. L. (2000). The mass media and the prevention of child behavior problems: The evaluation of a television series to promote positive outcomes for parents and their children. *Journal of Child Psychology and Psychiatry, 41*(7), 939–948. https://doi.org/10.1111/1469-7610.00681

Scarboro, M. E., & Forehand, R. (1975). Effects of two types of response-contingent time-out on compliance and oppositional behavior in children. *Journal of Experimental Child Psychology, 19*(2), 252–264. https://doi.org/10.1016/0022-0965(75)90089-2

Schreiber, M. E. (1999). Time-outs for toddlers: Is our goal punishment or education? *Young Children, 54*(4), 22–25.

Shriver, M. D., & Allen, K. D. (1996). The time-out grid: A guide to effective discipline. *School Psychology Quarterly, 11*(1), 67–74. https://doi.org/10.1037/h0088921

Sidman, M. (1989). *Coercion and its fallout*. Authors Cooperative.

Siegel, D. J. (2014, December 6). You said what about time-outs?! *Huffpost*. https://www.huffpost.com/entry/time-outs-overused_b_6006332

Siegel, D. J., & Bryson, T. P. (2014, September 23). Time-outs are hurting your child. *Time*. https://time.com/3404701/discipline-time-out-is-not-good/

Singh, N. N., & Katz, R. C. (1985). On the modification of acceptability ratings for alternative child treatments. *Behavior Modification, 9*(3), 375–386. https://doi.org/10.1177/01454455850093006

Skinner, B. F. (1950). Are theories of learning necessary? *Psychological Review, 57*(4), 193–216. https://doi.org/10.1037/h0054367

Skinner, B. F. (1953). *Science and human behavior*. MacMillan.

Society of Clinical Child and Adolescent Psychology (SCCAP). (2017). *Rule breaking, defiance, and acting out*. https://effectivechildtherapy.org/concerns-symptoms-disorders/disorders/rule-breaking-defiance-and-acting-out/

Solnick, J. V., Rincover, A., & Peterson, C. R. (1977). Some determinants of the reinforcing and punishing effects of timeout. *Journal of Applied Behavior Analysis, 10*(3), 415–424. https://doi.org.wvu.idm.oclc.org/10.1901/jaba.1977.10-415 https://doi.org/10.1901/jaba.1977.10-415

Solomon, R. L. (1964). Punishment. *American Psychologist, 19*(4), 239–253. https://doi.org/10.1037/h0042493

Solter, A. (1998). *Tears and tantrums: What to do when babies and children cry*. Shining Star Press/Aware Parenting Institute.

Staats, A. W. (1971). *Child learning, intelligence, and personality: Principles of a behavioral interaction approach*. Harper & Row.

Substance Abuse and Mental Health Services Administration. (2011). *Interventions for disruptive behavior disorders: Evidence-based and promising practices*. HHS Pub. No. SMA-11-4634. Center for Mental Health Services, SAMHSA, US Department of Health and Human Services. https://store.samhsa.gov/sites/default/files/d7/priv/sma11-4634-ebpspromisingpractices-idbd.pdf

Sue, D. W. (2004). Whiteness and ethnocentric monoculturalism: Making the "invisible" visible. *American Psychologist, 59*(8), 761–769. https://doi.org/10.1037/0003-066X.59.8.761

Taylor, J., & Miller, M. (1997). When timeout works some of the time: The importance of treatment integrity and functional assessment. *School Psychology Quarterly, 12*(1), 4–22. https://doi.org/10.1037/h0088943

The Incredible Years. (2013). *Time-out is one of many tools in the Incredible Years toolkit*. https://incredibleyears.com/parents-teachers/articles-for-teachers/

The MTA Cooperative Group. (1999). A 14-month randomized clinical trial of treatment strategies for attention-deficit/hyperactivity disorder. *Archives of General Psychiatry, 56*(12), 1073–1086. https://doi.org/10.1001/archpsyc.56.12.1073

Thompson, M. J. J., Laver-Bradbury, C., Ayres, M., le Poidevin, E., Mead, S., Dodds, C., Psychogiou, L., Bitsakou, P., Daley, D., Weeks, A., Miller Brotman, L., Abikoff, H., Thompason, P., & Sonuga-Barke, E. J. S. (2009). A small-scale randomized controlled trial of the revised new forest parenting programme for preschoolers with attention deficit hyperactivity disorder. *European Journal of Adolescent Psychiatry, 18*, 605-616. https://doi.org/10.1007/s00787-009-0020-0

Trentacosta, C. J., & Shaw, D. S. (2009). Emotional self-regulation, peer rejection, and antisocial behavior: Developmental associations from early childhood to early adolescence. *Journal of Applied Developmental Psychology, 30*(3), 356–365. https://doi.org/10.1016/j.appdev.2008.12.016

Turner, H. S., & Watson, T. S. (1999). Consultant's guide for the use of time-out in the preschool and elementary classroom. *Psychology in the Schools, 36*(2), 135–148. https://doi.org/10.1002/(SICI)1520-6807(199903)36:2<135::AID-PITS6>3.0.CO;2-3

Twyman, J. S., Johnson, H., Buie, J. D., & Nelson, M. (1994). The use of a warning procedure to signal a more intrusive timeout contingency. *Behavioral Disorders, 19*(4), 243–253. https://doi.org/10.1177/019874299401900407

Ucci, M. (1998). "Time outs" and how to use them. *Child Health Alert, 1*, 2–3.

Ulrich, R. E., & Azrin, N. H. (1962). Reflexive fighting in response to aversive stimulation. *Journal of the Experimental Analysis of Behavior, 5*(4), 511–520. https://doi.org/10.1901/jeab.1962.5-511

Ulrich, R. E., Wolff, P. C., & Azrin, N. H. (1964). Shock as an elicitor of intra- and interspecies fighting behavior. *Animal Behaviour, 12*(1), 14–15. https://doi.org/10.1016/0003-3472(64)90095-8

US Department of Education. (2010). *Summary of seclusion and restraint statutes, regulations, policies and guidance, by state and territory.* https://www2.ed.gov/policy/seclusion/seclusion-state-summary.html

Vander Schaaff, S. (2019, March 9). The man who developed timeouts for kids stands by his now hotly-debated idea. *The Washington Post.* https://www.washingtonpost.com/national/health-science/the-man-who-developed-timeouts-for-kids-stands-by-his-now-hotly-debated-idea/2019/03/08/c169439e-3159-11e9-8ad3-9a5b113ecd3c_story.html

Velasquez, L. D., Cathcart, A., Kennedy, A., & Allen, K. D. (2016). The effect of warnings to timeout on child compliance to parental instructions. *Child & Family Behavior Therapy, 38*(3), 225–244. https://doi.org/10.1080/07317107.2016.1203148

Wahler, R. G. (1969). Setting generality: Some specific and general effects of child behavior therapy. *Journal of Applied Behavior Analysis, 2*(4), 239–246. https://doi.org/10.1901/jaba.1969.2-239

Wang, M., & Kenny, S. (2014). Longitudinal links between fathers' and mothers' harsh verbal discipline and adolescents' conduct problems and depressive symptoms. *Child Development, 85*(3), 908–923. https://doi.org/10.1111/cdev.12143

Warzak, W. J., & Floress, M. T. (2009). Time-out training without put-backs, spanks, or restraint: A brief report of deferred time-out. *Child & Family Behavior Therapy, 31*(2), 134–143. https://doi.org/10.1080/07317100902910570

Webster-Stratton, C. (2001). The Incredible Years: Parents, teachers, and children training series. *Residential Treatment for Children & Youth, 18*(3), 31–45. https://doi.org/10.1300/J007v18n03_04

Webster-Stratton, C., & Reid, M. J. (2017). The Incredible Years parents, teachers, and children training series: A multifaceted treatment approach for young children with conduct problems. In J. R. Weisz & A. E. Kazdin (Eds.), *Evidence-based psychotherapies for children and adolescents* (3rd ed.; pp. 122–141). The Guilford Press.

Weeland, J., Chhangur, R. R., van der Giessen, D., Matthys, W., Orobio de Castro, B., & Overbeek, G. (2018). Intervention effectiveness of the Incredible Years: New insights into sociodemographic and intervention-based moderators: Corrigendum. *Behavior Therapy, 49*(2), 308–309. https://doi.org/10.1016/j.beth.2017.09.007

Whitacre, K. B., Foley, K., Jackson, C., Curtis, R., & McNeil, C. B. (2020). A comparison of Child Abuse Potential Inventory and Parenting Stress Index with families in the parent–child interaction therapy and treatment as usual groups. *Child & Family Behavior Therapy, 42*(3), 169–185. https://doi.org/10.1080/07317107.2020.1782005

White, G. D., Nielsen, G., & Johnson, S. M. (1972). Timeout duration and the suppression of deviant behavior in children. *Journal of Applied Behavior Analysis, 5*(2), 111–120. https://doi.org/10.1901/jaba.1972.5-111

Willoughby, R. H. (1970). The influence of different response consequences on children's preference for timeout. *Journal of Experimental Child Psychology, 9*(2), 133–141. https://doi.org/10.1016/0022-0965(70)90078-0

Wolf, M. M., Risley, T., & Mees, H. (1964). Application of operant conditioning procedures to the behaviour problems of an autistic child. *Behaviour Research and Therapy, 1*(2–4), 305–312. https://doi.org/10.1016/0005-7967(63)90045-7

Wolraich, M. L., Hagan, J. F., Jr., Allan, C., Chan, E., Davison, D., Earls, M., Evans, S. W., Flinn, S. K., Froehlich, T., Frost, J., Holbrook, J. R., Lehmann, C. U., Lessin, H. R., Okechukwu, K., Pierce, K. L., Winner, J. D., & Zurhellen, W. (2019). Clinical practice guideline for the diagnosis, evaluation, and treatment of attention-deficit/hyperactivity disorder in children and adolescents. *Pediatrics, 144*(4), Article e20192528. https://doi.org/10.1542/peds.2019-2528

Woodfield, M. J., Cargo, T., Barnett, D., & Lambie, I. (2020). Understanding New Zealand therapist experiences of parent–child interaction therapy (PCIT) training and implementation, and how these compare internationally. *Children and Youth Services Review, 119*, Article 105681. https://doi.org/10.1016/j.childyouth.2020.105681

12

Appendix: Tools and Resources

The materials on the following pages may be reproduced by the purchaser for personal/clinical use.
The printable, letter-sized PDFs can be downloaded free of charge from the Hogrefe website after registration.

Appendix 1: Useful Books and Websites for Parents and Caregivers
Appendix 2: Less Effective Versus More Effective Commands
Appendix 3: Parent–Child Interaction Therapy Compliance Training Time-Out: Follow-Through Diagrams
Appendix 4: Direct Commands Handouts

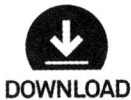

How to proceed:

1. Create a user account (or, if you have already one, please log in)

For customers from the USA, Canada, and the rest of the world:
hgf.io/login-us

For European customers:
hgf.io/login-eu

2. Download your supplementary materials

Go to **My supplementary materials** in your account dashboard and enter the code below. You will automatically be redirected to the download area, where you can access and download the supplementary materials.

Code: B-L8ITTC

To make sure you have permanent direct access to all the materials, we recommend that you download them and save them on your computer.

Appendix 1: Useful Books and Websites for Parents and Caregivers

Books

Barkley, R. A. (2013). *Your defiant child: Eight steps to better behavior* (2nd ed.). Guilford Press.

Clark, L. (2005). SOS: *Help for parents* (3rd ed.). SOS Programs & Parents Press.

Forehand, R., & Long, N. (2010). *Parenting the strong-willed child: The clinically proven five-week program for parents of two- to six-year-olds* (3rd ed.). McGraw Hill Professional.

Kazdin, A. E. (2008). *The Kazdin method for parenting the defiant child: With no pills, no therapy, no contest of wills.* Houghton Mifflin Company.

Webster-Stratton, C. (2019). *The Incredible Years: Trouble shooting guide for parents of children aged 3–8 years* (3rd ed.). The Incredible Years.

Websites

Centers for Disease Control and Prevention (CDC): Essentials for parenting toddlers and preschoolers.
https://www.cdc.gov/parents/essentials/index.html

Centers for Disease Control and Prevention (CDC): Guide to time-out.
https://www.cdc.gov/parents/essentials/timeout/handlingthings.html

Kazdin method: Online course "Everyday Parenting: The ABCs of Child Rearing."
https://www.coursera.org/learn/everyday-parenting

Parenting for Brain: Time out for kids – Correct steps and common mistakes.
https://www.parentingforbrain.com/time-out-for-toddler/

Triple P – Positive Parenting Program: Online course "Toddlers to Tweens."
https://www.triplep-parenting.com/us/get-started/online-parenting-course-toddlers-to-tweens/

See p. 110 for instructions on how to obtain the printable, letter-sized PDF.

Appendix 2: Less Effective Versus More Effective Commands

Less Effective	More Effective	Reason
• "Should I hold your coat?" • "Why don't you wipe your nose?" • "Want to hold my hand?"	• "Please, hand me your coat." • "Wipe your nose." • "Please, hold my hand."	More direct
• "Don't yell." • "Quit running." • "Stop hitting me."	• "Please, use a quiet voice." • "Walk." • "Put your hands in your lap, please."	Positively stated
• "Put on your shoes, coat, and backpack, and go to the car." • "Clean your room." • "Pick up, please."	• "Put on your shoes." • "Please, put your dirty clothes in the hamper." • "Put the pencils in this box, please."	One at a time
• "Act right." • "Settle down." • "Be careful."	• "Please, keep your hands to yourself." • "Sit next to me, please." • "Hold onto the railing."	More specific
• "Clean your room." (8-year-old) • "Go play with your Legos until dinner" (30 minutes). (5-year-old)	• "Please, put your books on the shelf." (8-year-old) • "Bring your Legos into the living room." (5-year-old)	More age/developmentally appropriate
• "I told you 100 times, stay in your seat!" • "Shut your mouth!" • "Give me the soda, right now!"	• "Sit in your chair, please." • "Please, whisper." • "Please, hand me the soda."	More polite and respectful
• "Turn off the movie, now." Child argues. • "It's almost bedtime." Child says they were just getting to the good part. • "You can watch for 5 more minutes." 5 minutes later child argues and refuses • "If you don't turn the movie off, there will be no movies tomorrow."	• **Before:** "It's almost bedtime. In 5 minutes, we'll need to turn off the movie." —5 minutes later— • **Command:** "Please, turn off the movie." —SILENCE— • **Compliance:** ✓ • **After:** "Thank you for listening. I know you were just getting to a good part, but we can watch a little in the morning because you listened so well."	Reasons and warnings are saved for <u>before</u> the command is given and/or <u>after</u> it is obeyed.

See p. 110 for instructions on how to obtain the printable, letter-sized PDF.

Appendix 3: Parent–Child Interaction Therapy Compliance Training Time-Out

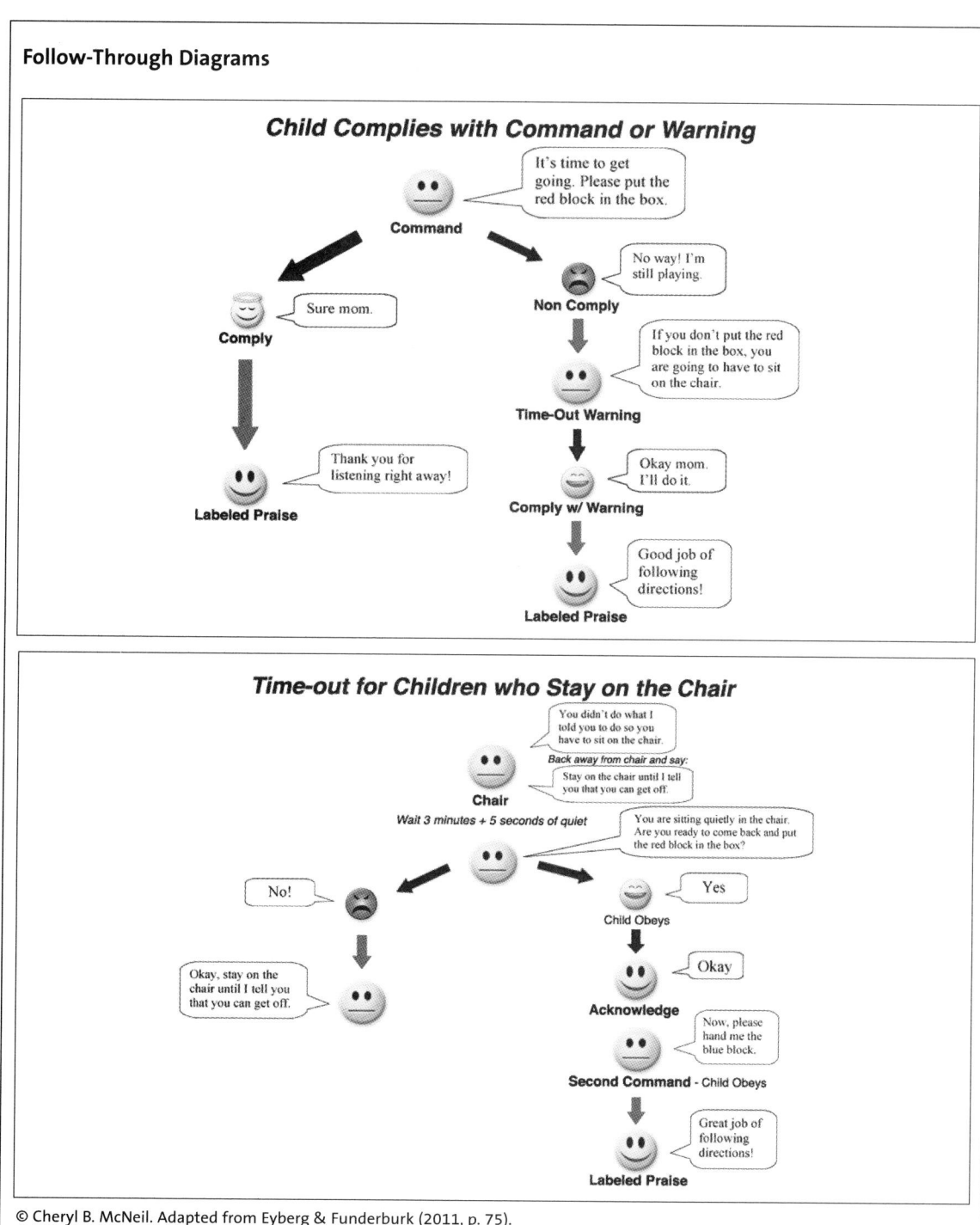

© Cheryl B. McNeil. Adapted from Eyberg & Funderburk (2011, p. 75).

See p. 110 for instructions on how to obtain the printable, letter-sized PDF.

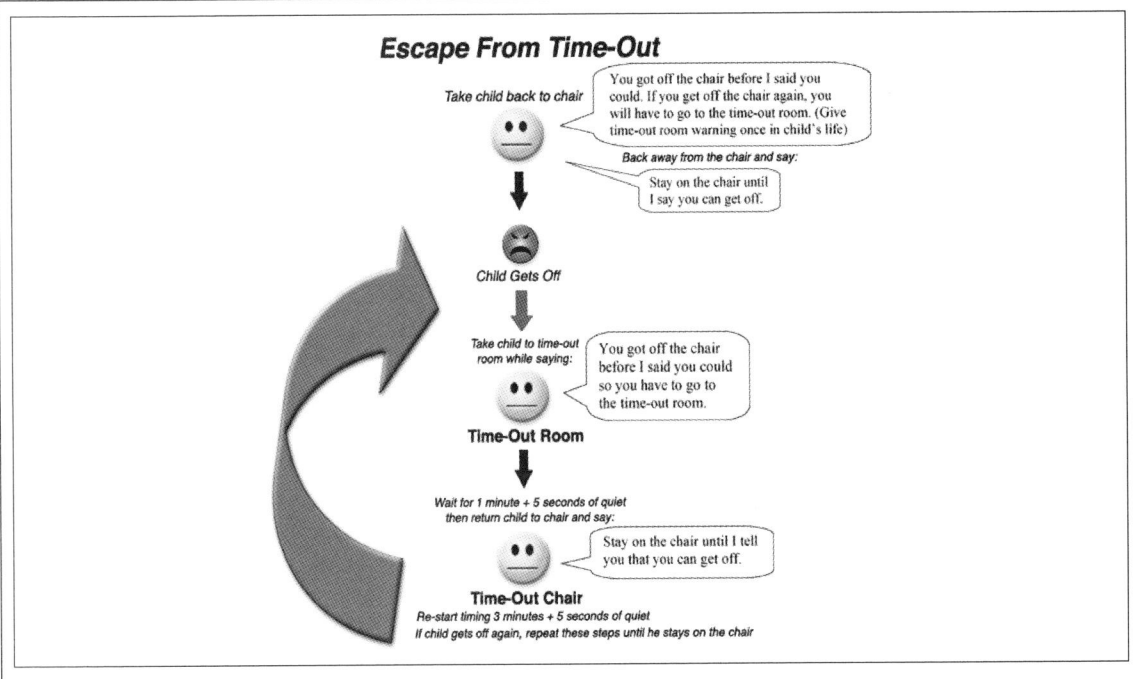

© Cheryl B. McNeil. Adapted from Eyberg & Funderburk (2011, p. 75).

Appendix 4: Direct Commands Handouts

Is This a Good Time for a Direct Command?

Consider the possibility that you may need to carry out a lengthy sequence including time-outs and trips to the back-up space if necessary.

The child must...	The caregiver must...	The environment must...
...be well-rested.	...have the time.	...have minimal distractions (siblings, screens, etc.).
...not be too hungry or thirsty.	...have the energy.	...be free of potential emergency and safety concerns (traffic, fire, water, spills, property damage).
...be alert.	...be calm.	...have a back-up space or alternative available.
...have recently used the toilet.	...be feeling well.	...have a clear path to the back-up space.
...be ready to learn. *Compliance training and time-out are opportunities to practice a new skill. Ask yourself if you would consider this an appropriate time to teach your child another new skill, for example, to write their name.*	...have patience and willingness in this moment to teach the child this new skill.	...have minimal potential for competing needs. *Ask yourself, am I in the middle of something (e.g., cooking) that will also require my attention? What will I do if the phone or doorbell rings?*
	...not have already given too many direct commands today. *Remember to pick your battles.*	...be free from others who may interfere with the procedure (e.g., co-parent, grandparent).

See p. 110 for instructions on how to obtain the printable, letter-sized PDF.

Alternatives to Direct Commands

These may be used when you have determined that now is NOT a good time for a direct command. Each option may be best suited for different situations and individual preferences.

Example: Your child walks into the house wearing muddy shoes. To address the situation, without giving a direct command (e.g., "Please, go back outside."), you could…

Strategy	Example
Use an indirect command	"Let's go back outside together."
DIY (Do It Yourself)	Take off the child's muddy shoes for them.
Physically guide	Carry the child to the bathtub.
Use child-directed interaction (CDI) skills	• Model taking off muddy shoes outside. • Model cleaning the floor and praise if the child starts to help. • Redirect with something exciting outside. • Ignore. • Ignore and praise the opposite (when child goes outside or takes off shoes).
Use logical consequences	Since you tracked mud on the floor, I would like you to help clean it up.
Use a "When…, then…" statement	"When you go back outside, then we can have a snack."
Structure the environment	Keep the door locked so the child cannot get into that room with muddy shoes.

See p. 110 for instructions on how to obtain the printable, letter-sized PDF.

Advances in Psychotherapy
Evidence-Based Practice

Developed and edited with the support of the Society of Clinical Psychology (APA Division 12)

Editor-in-chief
Danny Wedding, PhD, MPH

Associate editors
Jonathan S. Comer, PhD
Linda Carter Sobell, PhD, ABPP
Kenneth E. Freedland, PhD
J. Kim Penberthy, PhD, ABPP

- Practice-oriented
- Evidence-based
- Expert authors
- Easy-to-read
- Compact
- Cost-effective

Latest releases

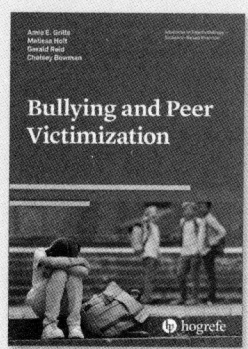

Volume 47
ISBN 978-0-88937-408-9

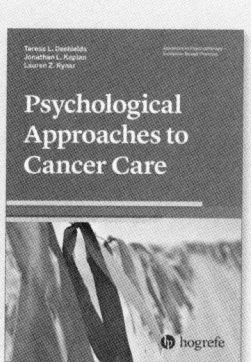

Volume 46
ISBN 978-0-88937-511-6

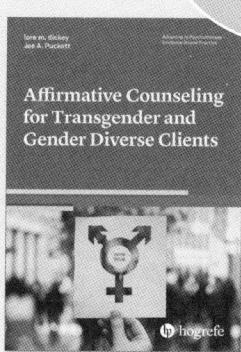

Volume 45
ISBN 978-0-88937-513-0

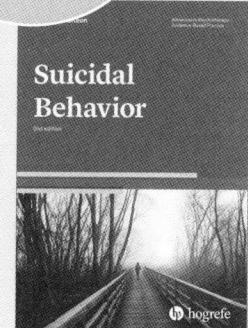

Volume 14, 2nd ed.
ISBN 978-0-88937-506-2

www.hogrefe.com

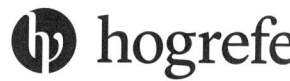

Advances in Psychotherapy
Evidence-Based Practice

All volumes of the series at a glance

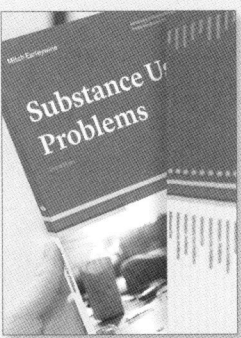

Affirmative Counseling for Transgender and Gender Diverse Clients (Vol. 45)
Alcohol Use Disorders (Vol. 10)
Alzheimer's Disease and Dementia (Vol. 38)
ADHD in Adults (Vol. 35)
ADHD in Children and Adolescents (Vol. 33)
Autism Spectrum Disorder (Vol. 29)
Binge Drinking and Alcohol Misuse Among College Students and Young Adults (Vol. 32)
Bipolar Disorder (Vol. 1, 2nd ed.)
Bullying and Peer Victimization (Vol. 47)
Body Dysmorphic Disorder (Vol. 44)
Childhood Maltreatment (Vol. 4, 2nd ed.)
Childhood Obesity (Vol. 39)
Chronic Illness in Children and Adolescents (Vol. 9)
Chronic Pain (Vol. 11)
Depression (Vol. 18)
Eating Disorders (Vol. 13)
Elimination Disorders in Children and Adolescents (Vol. 16)
Generalized Anxiety Disorder (Vol. 24)
Growing Up with Domestic Violence (Vol. 23)
Headache (Vol. 30)
Heart Disease (Vol. 2)
Hoarding Disorder (Vol. 40)
Hypochondriasis and Health Anxiety (Vol. 19)
Insomnia (Vol. 42)
Internet Addiction (Vol. 41)
Language Disorders in Children and Adolescents (Vol. 28)
Mindfulness (Vol. 37)
Multiple Sclerosis (Vol. 36)
Nicotine and Tobacco Dependence (Vol. 21)
Nonsuicidal Self-Injury (Vol. 22)
Obsessive-Compulsive Disorder in Adults (Vol. 31)
Persistent Depressive Disorders (Vol. 43)
Phobic and Anxiety Disorders in Children and Adolescents (Vol. 27)
Problem and Pathological Gambling (Vol. 8)
Psychological Approaches to Cancer Care (Vol. 46)
Public Health Tools for Practicing Psychologists (Vol. 20)
Sexual Dysfunction in Women (Vol. 25)
Sexual Dysfunction in Men (Vol. 26)
Sexual Violence (Vol. 17)
Social Anxiety Disorder (Vol. 12)
Substance Use Problems (Vol. 15, 2nd ed.)
Suicidal Behavior (Vol. 14, 2nd ed.)
The Schizophrenia Spectrum (Vol. 5, 2nd ed.)
Treating Victims of Mass Disaster and Terrorism (Vol. 6)
Women and Drinking: Preventing Alcohol-Exposed Pregnancies (Vol. 34)

Prices: US $29.80 / € 24.95 per volume. Standing order price US $24.80 / € 19.95 per volume (minimum 4 successive volumes) + postage & handling. Special rates for APA Division 12 and Division 42 members
Visit **hogrefe.com/us/apt** to get more information about the series!

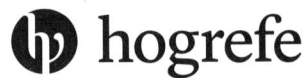

www.hogrefe.com